# Praise for *Wh[at Happens When] They Grow Up?*

"This book is for every mom who's spent years making sacrifices for their kids, and now worries about what happens when those years come to an end ... for every mom who is still waiting for 'someday' when she'll finally get everything done ... for every mom who wonders if anyone truly sees her. With her trademark wit and some very profound insights, Karen Johnson is the mom friend everyone needs to get through the trials that come with the territory."

—**Rita Templeton**, *Parenting Editor, SheKnows; former Deputy Editor of Scary Mommy*

"Motherhood, marriage, sacrifice ... the whole wad of adulting is in Karen Johnson's book, and it's exactly what you need to feel less alone."

—**Clint Edwards**, bestselling author of *Fatherish* and *Breaking Dad*

"As a middle-aged mother navigating the ever-evolving landscape of motherhood as my son grows up, I found myself deeply resonating with Karen's stories and insights. She beautifully explores the crossroads of motherhood and middle age, offering valuable guidance on how to navigate this new chapter—a time of rediscovery and reinvention beyond the role of 'snack-getter.'"

—**Tara Clark**, *founder, Modern Mom Probs*

# What Do I Want to Be When They Grow Up?

## (And Other Thoughts from a 40-Something Mom)

### Karen Johnson

**JOSSEY-BASS**
A Wiley Brand

Copyright © 2025 John Wiley & Sons, Inc. All rights, including for text and data mining, AI training, and similar technologies, are reserved.

Published by John Wiley & Sons, Inc., Hoboken, New Jersey.
Published simultaneously in Canada.

ISBNs: 9781394286300 (Paperback), 9781394286324 (ePDF), 9781394286317 (ePub).

No part of this publication may be reproduced, stored in a retrieval system, or transmitted in any form or by any means, electronic, mechanical, photocopying, recording, scanning, or otherwise, except as permitted under Section 107 or 108 of the 1976 United States Copyright Act, without either the prior written permission of the Publisher, or authorization through payment of the appropriate per-copy fee to the Copyright Clearance Center, Inc., 222 Rosewood Drive, Danvers, MA 01923, (978) 750-8400, fax (978) 750-4470, or on the web at www.copyright.com. Requests to the Publisher for permission should be addressed to the Permissions Department, John Wiley & Sons, Inc., 111 River Street, Hoboken, NJ 07030, (201) 748-6011, fax (201) 748-6008, or online at http://www.wiley.com/go/permission.

Trademarks: Wiley and the Wiley logo are trademarks or registered trademarks of John Wiley & Sons, Inc. and/or its affiliates in the United States and other countries and may not be used without written permission. All other trademarks are the property of their respective owners. John Wiley & Sons, Inc. is not associated with any product or vendor mentioned in this book.

Limit of Liability/Disclaimer of Warranty: While the publisher and author have used their best efforts in preparing this book, they make no representations or warranties with respect to the accuracy or completeness of the contents of this book and specifically disclaim any implied warranties of merchantability or fitness for a particular purpose. No warranty may be created or extended by sales representatives or written sales materials. The advice and strategies contained herein may not be suitable for your situation. You should consult with a professional where appropriate. Further, readers should be aware that websites listed in this work may have changed or disappeared between when this work was written and when it is read. Neither the publisher nor authors shall be liable for any loss of profit or any other commercial damages, including but not limited to special, incidental, consequential, or other damages.

For general information on our other products and services or for technical support, please contact our Customer Care Department within the United States at (800) 762-2974, outside the United States at (317) 572-3993 or fax (317) 572-4002.

Wiley also publishes its books in a variety of electronic formats. Some content that appears in print may not be available in electronic formats. For more information about Wiley products, visit our web site at www.wiley.com.

*Library of Congress Control Number:* 2025000806 (print)

Cover Design: Paul McCarthy
Cover Photo: Courtesy of Karen Johnson

SKY10100503_031925

*To eight-year-old me, handwriting books in her bedroom
and binding them together with twine,
telling everyone,
"I'm going to be a writer someday"…
We did it. I'm proud of us.*

# Contents

Prologue ix

**Chapter 1:** What Do I Want to Be When They Grow Up? 1
**Chapter 2:** Guilt 11
**Chapter 3:** You Can't Do It All, So Quit Trying 17
**Chapter 4:** When Mothers Are Ghosts 25
**Chapter 5:** How Much Are SAHMs Actually Worth? 29
**Chapter 6:** The Default Parenting Ferris Wheel 35
**Chapter 7:** That Day I Hiked 14 Miles and Braced for a Hip Replacement (But Also Realized Something about Me as a Mom) 41
**Chapter 8:** "Hi, I'm Sweating!" (WTF Is Happening to My Body?) 49
**Chapter 9:** On Aging and Beauty Culture (So, I Guess I Have a Turkey Neck Now...? Whatever) 57
**Chapter 10:** On Friendships 63
**Chapter 11:** The Comparison Trap 69

| | | |
|---|---|---|
| **Chapter 12:** | The Water Challenge (and How We Need to Reframe "Success") | 77 |
| **Chapter 13:** | Get Thee to a Therapist! | 81 |
| **Chapter 14:** | Of Course We're Pissed Off | 89 |
| **Chapter 15:** | Anxiety, Perfectionism, + a Crippling Fear of Failure = a Toxic Cocktail that Does Not Mix with Motherhood | 95 |
| **Chapter 16:** | Learning to Get Out of My Own Way | 103 |
| **Chapter 17:** | Nobody Talks About the Loneliness | 109 |
| **Chapter 18:** | How Resentment and the "Who Has It Harder" Game Nearly Killed My Marriage, and the Daily Phone Call That Probably Saved It | 119 |
| **Chapter 19:** | Lessons for My Kids (and for Myself) as We All Grow Up | 127 |
| **Chapter 20:** | The Death of Martyrdom | 135 |
| **Chapter 21:** | "Everything Is Fine," "I Don't Care What Other People Think," and Other Lies We Tell | 141 |
| **Chapter 22:** | How I "Lost Myself" but Found the Pieces and Put Myself Back Together | 151 |
| **Chapter 23:** | How Did I Get Here? (The Story of Our Gladiator Turtles, Medically Fragile Dog, and One Dead Plant) | 159 |
| **Chapter 24:** | The Many Forms of Motherhood Grief | 165 |
| **Chapter 25:** | Always Awkward, Never Cool | 171 |
| **Chapter 26:** | Halfway There (and Livin' on a Prayer) | 177 |
| **Chapter 27:** | Make Me a Promise | 185 |
| **Chapter 28:** | I'm a Total Fraud (by the Way) | 193 |
| **Chapter 29:** | We Can Do Hard Things (and Let Me Tell You How I Know) | 197 |
| **Chapter 30:** | So, What AM I Going to Be When They Grow Up? | 203 |

| | |
|---|---|
| Epilogue | 207 |
| Acknowledgments | 209 |
| About the Author | 211 |

# Prologue

I don't like surprises. I mean, of course I like the good kind like when my husband proposed in our tiny apartment kitchen a hundred years ago and I was utterly, entirely shocked. That kind I love. LOVE. But as a type-A anxiety-ridden perfectionist, I like having a plan. I like knowing what's coming next. And I like being prepared. The word "spontaneity" doesn't really get much usage in my world. But there have been two times in my life when a major life change hit hard and the ground under me shifted, like an earthquake that threw everything off kilter.

Unsteady ground? Don't like it. 0/10. Do not recommend.

The first time I felt one of those unwelcome surprises was when I became a mom. The "becoming a mom" part was beautiful and exactly what I wanted—that wasn't the shock. It was everything else: the loneliness, the isolation, the abrupt shift of leaving my career, the feelings of failure and staring at the clock, counting the minutes and hours until I'd see another adult.

I was not on steady ground, and I didn't know what to do.

The second time I felt the whiplash of a "Whoa, I did not see that coming" event was as I entered all the sweaty glory of perimenopause. I did not know my body would change so drastically and so fast, and I have to say this has also been a very unwelcome surprise. Also 0/10. Zero stars.

But now another big one is heading my way and maybe heading your way, too. Yet another major life change is on the horizon as our little kids have grown into big kids and are starting to strengthen their wings so they can fly off in the near future.

So, I've decided to be prepared—as best I can. I'm learning about myself so I know what I need (and will need) as a woman, a wife, a mom, and a writer. I'm self-reflecting about why I have struggled in the past and thinking about what I can do in the future to solidify myself in solid ground. And I'm writing this book to share my thoughts so that maybe I can help you prepare a little bit, too.

*So yes, if you're a woman, this book is for you.*

*If you're a mom, this book is for you.*

*If you're a perfectionist or if you have anxiety (or if you're a perfectionist WITH anxiety—yay for you by the way), this book is for you.*

Also, this book is for anyone out there who:

*Gave up their career to raise their kids.*

*Is the default parent.*

*Is in the throes of perimenopause (or really just wants to read about how super fun it is!)*

*Is a little (or a lot) pissed off about, well, everything. (Let's be pissed off together!)*

*Has ever driven their pet turtle to the vet in a Tupperware bowl. (That's weirdly specific, but yes, there's a chapter on our high-need pets.)*

*Has neck, arm, and eyelid skin that is getting looser and wrinklier because they're, well, aging (like everyone else).*

*Has felt grief and regret that in some ways, motherhood didn't turn out like it was supposed to.*

*And finally, if you're just the kind of person who wants to read someone else's real, honest, raw stories about being a mom and navigating life and trying to figure out what she's going to do when the kids aren't around anymore to beg for takeout or fight over having to walk the dog, this book is absolutely for you.*

The stories in this book are true. They're mine. I share them with you as a series of tiny therapy sessions (for you and for me) and also to hopefully make you laugh and feel less alone. And maybe, if we all do it together, we can learn to unapologetically just *like* ourselves—how great would that be?

We're all in this sweaty-perimenopausal-what's-next-for-me time of life together. I know I need girlfriends to get through it, and maybe you do too. Thanks for reading and for being here.

—Karen
(The 21st Century SAHM)

# Chapter 1

# What Do I Want to Be When They Grow Up?

I'm a planner. (Shocking, right, when you see that I have a whole chapter in this book dedicated to anxiety and perfectionism.) And in the summer of 2008, I had a plan for exactly how life was going to go. Glowing and pregnant with my first child, I was also on the cusp of a big change professionally. Not necessarily because of the baby who'd soon be joining our family, but because my husband and I were planning a move (from Wisconsin to Kansas) for his job. I was an English teacher at the time, so the summer months were the perfect time for me to visit Kansas, tour potential high schools, and meet some principals, hoping to make a connection and land a new job myself. And, while we were there, we checked out neighborhood options, as well.

I had it all mapped out. I'd get a new job as a teacher, be a working mom who brought her kid to daycare or had a nanny, and we'd likely live in a bungalow-style house, near Kansas City, where we could raise our little baby in an eclectic and vibrant community full of quaint bakeries, botanical gardens, and libraries we could walk to on Saturdays.

Boom. Plan.

Except none of that happened.

In reality, my story followed the path of so many women with lofty ambitions to do it all and have it all. And then, at some point, reality smacks them in the face with a sippy cup full of day-old milk and they realize they can't.

## The Best Laid Plans ...

So, what happened? Why didn't I end up heading the English department at a high school in Kansas and walk my baby to the farmers market on Saturday mornings?

I MEAN, I HAD A PLAN.

Was it because I hated my job? Nope. I loved teaching. Absolutely loved it. Also, I had already earned my undergraduate and master's degrees in English and Secondary Teaching. Why wouldn't I continue working in a career I was passionate about? A career I was really freaking good at? A career I'd be paying for until I was in my 40s (because, you know, student loans and all)?

Why did I walk away? Why do so many of us women who love our careers—careers we worked our asses off for—walk away as we pivot into motherhood? And why is it usually us doing it and not the dads?

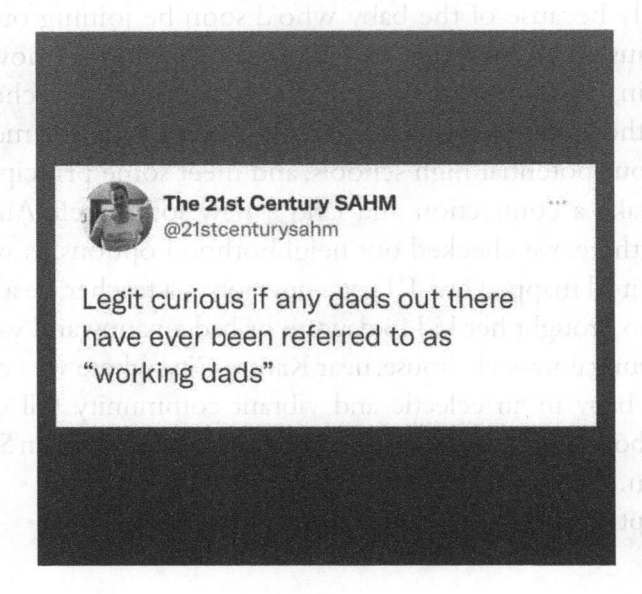

> **The 21st Century SAHM**
> @21stcenturysahm
>
> Legit curious if any dads out there have ever been referred to as "working dads"

(You're probably expecting an answer here, but I don't have one.)

For me, there was no aha moment when a light switch flipped and I knew my teaching career was over. But sometime after my baby was born, my husband and I were standing in our tiny apartment kitchen, and he looked at me and said, "You're not going back to teaching, are you?"

He knew. He was right. And that was that.

Maybe it was due to the mom in me emerging and finding myself pulled to cul-de-sac neighborhoods with minivans rather than the urban downtown vibe I thought I wanted.

Maybe it was because almost immediately after starting his new job, my husband began traveling often, and I knew the only way I could teach high school English was if I dropped my tiny little baby off at a daycare at 6:30 in the morning.

Or maybe it was because I was, frankly, overwhelmed by motherhood and knew with my whole heart that I'd never again be able to give myself to teaching in the way I used to.

Honestly, it was likely a combination of all of these, but yes, that was the end. I never got my teaching license in Kansas and never went back to the classroom after we moved.

My first child was still an infant, and my teaching days were done.

Sixteen years later, I still refer to myself as a former teacher and I still treasure those seven years in the classroom as one of the most important times in my life.

But it's true—instead of teaching Shakespearean sonnets and the value of a good transition between paragraphs, I've spent the last decade and a half changing diapers, attending play dates, reading animal farm books, potty-training three kids, washing straws, lids, and endless tiny cups, building Lego sets, and sweeping crumbs off the floor.

It's been a beautiful, messy, exhausting ride, but the reality is that throughout parenthood, my two college degrees have merely collected dust while my husband's career flourished.

It was a choice I made—a choice I 100% do not regret and I fully believe was the best option for me at the time—but it changed the entire trajectory of my life. I never imagined before becoming pregnant that the end of my time in the classroom was near, and then, suddenly it was.

## The Default Parent Uber Driver Life

My youngest is now 12. The others are 14 and 16. They're in school all day long, which leaves lots of quiet hours for me and the dog. I've been freelancing as a writer and editor since the second baby arrived, so I've got something (a lot, actually) to show for myself when it comes to "work" and that awkward question SAHMs often get that makes us twitch with rage: *So what do you DO all day?"*

But no, it's not a full-time job. There's no office holiday party or retirement fund or health insurance. I swap in one pair of sweats for another, throw in a load of laundry, do a little work, take the dog for a walk, make sure dinner is prepped for later, put the laundry in the dryer, run the dishwasher, register a kid for something, make an appointment for another, rinse and repeat. Day after day.

During the school year, the high schoolers arrive home at around 3:15, the tween at 4:25. By 5:00, I'm in the car almost every day, driving them all over town to practice, rehearsal, a game, or a friend's house and often don't come up for air until many hours later.

It's not a bad gig. In fact, I'm quite blessed to be the one there for everything, the one absorbing all the car ride convos where bits of information leak out, the one helping edit essays and quizzing them on vocab, the one helping them navigate friendship woes and cheering them on at every game, show, or competition they throw themselves into.

But now that I'm less than a decade from the last one moving on to a post-high-school life, I do wonder ... What do I want to be when they grow up? Is this it? Freelancing, still doing the laundry, and walking the dog every day at noon? Is that enough? Do *I* want a turn at a thriving, booming career like my husband has had? Do I want a big retirement bash like he'll have someday? Do I want a justified reason to actually wear real pants once in a while?

Are these even options for me?

Knowing that, as the default parent, I'm endlessly on standby for:

"*Mom, can you bring me ____ (insert book, computer, phone, charger, uniform, food, etc. etc., forever and ever, amen)*" …

Or "*Mom, I don't feel well. Can you pick me up?*" …

Or "*Mom, my game is an hour away so we need to leave right after school to get there on time*"…

I know that any steady "job" or career aspiration, at least for now, has to fit snugly between the 8:30 and 3:00 hours. And that I have to be able and willing to respond and possibly hop into my car on a moment's notice during those hours too.

Of course, kids with moms who work full-time survive and thrive even if their mother can't appear like a magician with whatever they forgot at home. But because my husband works long hours and sometimes travels, the after-school-driving-all-over-the-state part of my job … that one's here to stay for a few more years, so I'd have to find a career that frees up when the kids do.

But wait! I do have those two degrees taking up space in the hall closet!

"*What about teaching?*" people sometimes ask. "*Why don't you return to the classroom?*" And to be honest, I don't fully know the answer to why that's a "No" for me, but I think it's a swirl of factors. Career fields go through monumental change in a decade's time, and that's how long it was until my third and last baby was in school. By 2018, the landscape of teaching looked completely different from anything I'd known. When I left the field in 2009, most of my students didn't even have cell phones yet. No one had a smartphone. I can't imagine time-hopping all these years and adjusting to what a classroom full of adolescents looks like now.

Also, I graded papers every night, every weekend, back in my pre-kid 20s. Those hours are gone now, entirely consumed with my own children. Sure, lots of moms do it—I have several friends who remained in the classroom, raised their own kids, and are badass teacher-moms who make it all work. For me, it's too much. I never gave myself the chance to evolve, to share the mental load with my husband, to learn what it looks like to manage mom life and teacher life simultaneously. Re-entering the teacher workforce today feels like diving head-first into a pit of lava.

I believe I'd be setting myself on a straight path to overwhelming failure—a path where as I'd feared all those years ago, I'd be doing two jobs, and neither of them well.

I've spent my children's entire lives as their default parent. I've been there for every need, every call from the nurse, every snow day, every school event. And any parent with older kids knows that even when they are big enough to go off to school all day long, the needs don't stop. How could I possibly make the shift to going back to work full-time? Our system has worked for the last 16 years because my husband cannot be on standby, whereas I can. I am the stable, stationary one who is always home. Always there. They rely on that—him and the kids. And, to be honest, I love being that person for all four of them.

And finally, I guess I just see those seven years as a wholly separate chapter in my story. I loved the teacher I was, and I want to preserve that memory. I can't ever be her again—completely and utterly devoted to her career and her career only. Those seven years are preserved, almost as if they are in a snow globe, untouchable, sitting on a shelf, bringing back memories and making me smile with pride at the time I taught *Hamlet* and *To Kill a Mockingbird* in another life.

## Scared to Try, Scared to Not Try

What is next, then? I have six years until my last baby leaves for college. And as much as I want to chase my dreams and toss my hat into the ring of ... something, if I'm being honest, I'm also terrified.

I'm scared to put myself out there What does that other world full of "career people" even look like? Is there even a place for me anymore?

But if I don't try, then what? And that's the scariest question of all.

For now, here I am, in the middle. My kids are all in school full-time, but I'm still the default parent they call for everything. Every third Wednesday is a half-day of school, so I that's when I schedule orthodontist appointments and usually try to fit in another errand like haircuts, as well. Right now we're out of eggs and cheese, so I'm going to run to the grocery store real quick for a few things, and, while I'm out, I'll pop into Kohl's and grab new sneakers for my oldest, whose feet won't stop growing, and oh yeah, I need to refill the dog's medicine, too.

And that's why so many of us slog through the grueling baby and toddler days only to emerge on the other side when all the kids are in school, wondering what we should do with ourselves now. Except we're still the household managers with nine thousand tiny but very important tasks to manage daily, and we have to be at the front of the car line to get the youngest one to practice on time, so we actually have to leave the house at 2:45.

*Teacher, writer, mom, wife.* These are the various maps by which I've lived my life. For now, and for the past decade and a half, "*Mom*" tends to be the compass and everything else falls into place around it.

After another 16 years? I might have a different compass or a new map. Maybe I'll have real-life coworkers and a reason to wear pants that button. Or maybe this is it forever and I'm Team Sweatpants for life.

I don't know yet. For now, I guess I'll go throw in a load of towels while I keep wondering what comes next.

## Notes on Chapter 1

*If this story sounds familiar to you, you might also be wondering what you're going to be when they grow up. So, as you muddle through these middle years, remember these three things:*

- First of all, (and most importantly), if you want your life to include more than motherhood, that's nothing to feel guilty about. You're a great mom and it's okay to want more because you deserve it. Write that on a Post-it and stick it to your mirror.
- Secondly, the time to start prioritizing yourself is now (like yesterday, actually). This way, when the house is actually quiet in a few years, you've already taken a few steps toward your new, well, "you." That means giving real, meaningful thought to what you're passionate about. What parts of you lay hidden all these years because motherhood consumed your every waking breath?
- Also, if you wonder if you're qualified to put yourself out there, remember that through motherhood, you've done a million jobs you had no training for, but you figured it out. As moms, we multitask, run a household, manage calendars and schedules for multiple people, meal-plan and cook to meet different dietary needs, and field punches on the daily in the form of emotional meltdowns, failed tests, and friendship drama, just to name a few. And that's just on a Tuesday.

**There's nothing you can't do.**

But if you're stuck, here are some ideas. I have lots of friends in the same boat as us—with older kids who have flown the coop or are about to—and here's what they're doing:

1. Going back to school. New degree, new me!
2. Starting their own small businesses, selling their own unique creations, like custom-made clothes.

3. Marketing their services—things they're good at—home organization, cleaning services, photography, personal assistant work.
4. Pivoting career paths entirely and putting themselves out there to do a job they've never done before. They just knew they'd be good at it, so they aimed high and landed the role.
5. Joining the real estate business and killing it.
6. Flipping houses. (Fingers crossed they'll help me redo mine.)
7. Dusting off that old degree, but taking it in a different direction. Former teachers are subbing, tutoring, and teaching online school. Friends who used to work in marketing are reaching out to local businesses to see who needs help getting the word out on social media.
8. Opening up their homes to in-home daycare for little ones.
9. Training to become foster parents as they know their home is meant to have kids running through it, and they felt a calling to help kids who need some love and stability.
10. And me? Well, looks like I'm writing a book.

The truth is, that next chapter is coming, whether you want it to or not. Someday they will all grow up. So what are you going to be?

# Chapter 2

# Guilt

In childhood, it was a new friend. We didn't know better, so we welcomed Guilt into our circle, not knowing how fast this frenemy was sadistically worming its way into our psyche.

*When you accidentally broke the vase at Grandma's ...*

*When you talked out of turn at school and received a glare from the teacher ...*

*When you stained your new dress with spaghetti sauce even though you promised to be extra careful ...*

It's not hard to train young children to accept Guilt into their innocent little lives.

By the teen and young adult years, we were well acquainted, as Guilt had shown itself now quite a bit over the years—always there, looming, lurking, fully seeped into our subconscious where it had grown roots—first a tree, then a forest.

That boy who likes you and is in your personal space? *"Be nice or you'll hurt his feelings,"* Guilt said.

Don't want to take that extra shift at work? *"But your boss really needs you to come in, even though you were supposed to have today off. He's short-staffed!"* Guilt told you.

*"Don't eat that piece of cake. You didn't work out this morning,"* Guilt whispered in our ear, over and over.

## How Guilt Creates the Zombie Mom

Knowing this history, it's not surprising that Mom Guilt is so pervasive, such a powerful force in our well-being (or lack thereof) as we navigate the journey of child-raising.

Mom Guilt is just a spawn of something that's already been there for as long as we can remember.

But once you're holding that tiny baby in your arms, Guilt and all its spiky tentacles takes on new forms, grows new roots, and finds new corners of your mind to sink its teeth into.

Working mom?

*"How could you leave your child in the care of someone else?"*

Stay-at-home mom?

*"Why are you wasting your college degree? What do you do all day?"* *"Why are your kids watching screens and not playing outside right now?"*

Missed "Muffins with Mom" at your child's preschool?

*"Wow. All the other moms were there."*

Not volunteering at school?

*"Hmmm. Thankfully other moms care enough to help out."*

House isn't clean?

*"Get it together."*

Haven't showered or done your makeup or hair in days?

*"Do you even try? What does your husband think?"*

Gained weight?

*"You really should make time to work out, eat healthier, lose the 'baby weight,' practice self-care."*

Child misbehaves?

*"Why aren't you disciplining them?"*

Kids eat junk food?

*"Don't you even care what goes into your child's body?"*

Looking at your phone and not at your child every second?

*"Why did you even have kids?!"*

And it grows stronger and stronger.

If our teens struggle with mental health issues, *we blame ourselves.*

If we lose a pregnancy, *we blame ourselves*.

If our kids get sick or get hurt, *we blame ourselves*.

Mom Guilt is the loudest and the strongest of all the Guilts, isn't it?

That's because Mom Guilt partners up with that dangerous *"You can do it all!"* mindset and together, they set you up for complete and utter failure. And it's because of Mom Guilt that there's a sea of exhausted zombie moms shuffling through the halls at parent-teacher conferences. Moms who have been up since 5 a.m., have already worked a full day, have dinner cooking in the crockpot, and need to rush home after meeting with the math teacher (*"How can I get him to practice his math facts more?"* you'll ask, feeling guilty when you look at his test scores) and ensure the soccer uniform is washed—three games this weekend! You'll be there! Good moms are prepared and have healthy meals ready and uniforms washed. Their houses are clean and their kids are all well-adjusted and have all their needs met and see their mom at every single game, play, musical, band concert ... Good moms don't miss a beat, right?

You know those guilt-ridden zombie moms at school events (maybe you are one).

Zombie Mom carries a water bottle that she'll accidentally leave on one of the children's desks at open house meet-the-teacher night. (She's trying and failing to drink more water—you know, *self-care*.)

Zombie Mom will notice that the signup sheet for "room parent" or "book fair volunteer" still has open slots and despite her sheer exhaustion and having zero idea how she'll find time to squeeze more responsibilities into her life, she jots down her name next to the other moms. There aren't nearly as many dads on the list, nor are there as many dads roaming the halls at conferences, bracing for the next teacher assessment about reading scores. (*"Is he doing his nightly reading?"* the teacher will ask Zombie Mom, with a disappointed tone.)

## Mom Guilt vs. Dad Guilt

So, how does the guilt-ridden Zombie Mom form? Why do we always take on more even though we're at capacity?

Is it because of that nagging voice we've been hearing since we were children about never being good enough, never being allowed to say "no" or else we'd hurt someone's feelings, never letting anyone down or else we weren't good people? Has Guilt not been living with dads since they were boys? Did they get through adolescence and adulthood without its constant presence? Is Dad Guilt quieter or weaker, or are they just better equipped at fending it off?

I'm sure dads feel guilty in lots of ways, just like moms do. And a lot of the dads in my life are the hardest working, most loving, dedicated fathers on the planet. But they do seem to have an easier time ignoring that volunteer signup sheet or going to sleep if the house is a mess.

Also, maybe because society doesn't say, "*How could you possibly let someone else raise your kids?*" to working dads, then Dad Guilt isn't whispering it in their ear as they head off to work or take that promotion.

Maybe because no one at the park judges the dad for looking at his phone and, in fact, praises him as Dad of the Year for even packing up the kids and taking them out of the house at all. Maybe, that's why Dad Guilt just isn't as powerful.

Or because when Dad gives his kid candy and lets the kids skip reading homework, he's the "fun dad!" but when Mom does it, she's neglectful.

And when Dad's body changes as he ages, he's got a "hot dad bod" but Mom (who *actually gave birth*) is "letting herself go."

Guilt tells us we shouldn't want more out of our careers because what kind of mother would we be? But does Guilt say that to dads?

For our whole lives, Guilt tells us we're too fat, too loud, and too much, but also not enough all in one vindictive whisper in our ear.

The truth is, girlfriends, we let Guilt have too much power. We let it tell us that we need to do all the things and be at all the events and never waver, not even for a second, even though we're running on our very last drop after managing the mental load Ferris wheel 24/7 for the past decade (see Chapter 6).

*We cannot be too tired*, Guilt says. *We cannot be too busy. We cannot forget anything.*

Unfortunately though, moms often don't win in the end. Guilt wins because we're dead in the ground having run ourselves into martyrdom (see Chapter 20), having put ourselves last, having desperately tried to quiet the toxic whispers we've been hearing since we were kids.

### Screw You, Guilt. I'm Eating the Cake.

But what if we're not willing to accept that sad ending? What if it's time we stop letting Guilt—specifically Mom Guilt—win the war? What would that look like? It might look like walking past the volunteer signup sheet because you just can't take on one more thing right now. It might look like prioritizing your career now, and letting your kids see what it looks like when Mom puts herself first because she's waited a long time and deserves a shot.

It might look like eating cake, because cake is delicious, and not tying a dessert to whether you've worked out or not.

It might look like accepting that you're aging, you're tired, your house isn't clean, but you're doing your damn best and you sit down with a glass of wine, ignore the laundry pile, and flip on Netflix, drowning out Guilt with the sounds of binge-watching your favorite show and slowly sipping a glass of Merlot.

## Notes on Chapter 2

*Okay, so how DO we effectively beat Guilt at its game? Try these three steps:*

1. **Stop "should-ing" yourself.**

    When you hear it happening in your head: "I should work out, I shouldn't eat this piece of pizza, I should lose weight, I should clean the house more, I should, I should, I should…"

    Should-ing yourself is just sprinkling extra shame all over the parts of motherhood and life where you feel inadequate. And shame is toxic and harmful. If you want to regularly eat healthy, work out, have a cleaner house, etc., those are all healthy goals if you're doing them for the right reasons. Make a realistic schedule or plan to achieve them, and if it doesn't work out today (or tomorrow, or the next day), try again or reevaluate your schedule. But working your tail off all day to be everything for everyone and then should-ing yourself into a feeling of failure rather than priding yourself in how much you did do doesn't serve you in any way.

2. **Practice self-compassion.**

    Okay, so you missed your kid's big home run the other night or you snapped at your spouse for leaving his shoes by the door where everyone can trip over them. You feel like utter crap, but you're not a bad mom or spouse or a bad person at all. You're a human. You're doing your best. And you deserve kindness, forgiveness, and grace, especially from yourself.

3. **Be on your own side.**

    That means focusing on things you like about yourself—write them down on a Post-it. Stick them to your mirror. Write them in your journal. Say them out loud. What makes you a good mom? What makes you a good friend? What makes you a good partner in life? Are you kind? Funny? Creative? Unique? Devoted? Loving? Hardworking? Don't let Guilt win and tell you otherwise.

# Chapter 3

# You Can't Do It All, So Quit Trying

I remember when my kids were babies and toddlers and our days were spent playing pretend "store" and stacking wooden letter blocks ... maybe going outside to look for pretty leaves or drawing with sidewalk chalk. I felt like during those years, I was always doing laundry—so many tiny socks. I was always picking up toys and putting them back into bins. And I was always, *always* emptying the dishwasher, reloading the dishwasher, and emptying it again, letting rows and rows of plastic sippy cups air-dry all over my kitchen counter because no matter what "drying cycle" I tried on that damn thing, those little cups were never ever dry.

I remember spending my days looking around the room, looking around my house, and thinking "*Someday. Someday, they'll all be in school and I'll finally have time to get everything done. I'll finally have a clean house and have the meals cooked and the groceries bought and the laundry done. And I'll have time for me! I'll work out! I'll read books! Oh, the books I'll read,*" I thought. "*And I'll drink lots of water, not just coffee all day long, and I'll finally be one of those put-together moms who blow-dries her hair and wears eye makeup more than once a month.*"

"*Someday,*" I thought.

Well, someday arrived. At least in the sense that my children did grow up to become older kids who go to school full-time. But that's pretty much it for the rest of that story. It's a decade later. Those babies and toddlers are now in middle and high school. I don't spend my days playing pretend "store" anymore, and the wooden blocks have long since been donated to other families with tiny hands and curious little minds just learning their letters. But somehow, I'm still always doing laundry. Only instead of piles upon piles of tiny socks, I just wash piles upon piles of bigger, stinkier socks. And no, the dishes still aren't done. There are still cups everywhere, always air-drying on my kitchen counter. We still run out of food we need, and the meals are rarely prepared when we need them to be.

And now that "someday" is here, I've come to realize something. I have spent the past 10–15 years dreaming of the day when I could look around at my life and say, "*I did it! I did all the things today! I can do it all.*"

I've spent years dreaming of something that will never ever come true.

The truth is, I can't do it all. And you know what? Neither can you.

Not because you're a failure. Not because I'm a failure. But because we have two arms. And two legs. And 24 hours in a day. And seven days in a week. And we have to sleep (at least a little).

The thing is, we grew up in a tricky generation. We were fed a lot of bullshit lines about having it all, doing it all. We were built up to believe in ourselves: "*There's nothing girls can't do!*" And it's true. We *can* do anything. Our daughters can do anything. And I love that we absorbed that message and believed in ourselves and I've passed it wholeheartedly onto my teenage daughter all her life.

But the thing is, although we *can* do *anything*, we *can't* do it *all*—at least, not all at once.

And that's the part of the story we were missing. No one told us that if you want to do one really huge, awesome thing that you're proud of, that you might not be able to do this other really huge, awesome thing you'd also be proud of at the exact same time, or as well as you've done the first thing (because, again, two arms, two legs, 24 hours, seven days).

No one told us that, so we all grew up believing a lie.

And now we're moms in our 40s and we're trying to actually, literally, do it all.

We're kicking ass at careers that we deserve! Go us! But we're also still totally hands-on moms who don't miss a beat! And we're working out, getting back into shape after having babies because we aren't frumpy moms! We'll work out at 4 a.m. since that's the only hour left!

We're ... doing ... it ... all ... (cue us all breathless and falling off a cliff of exhaustion).

Because we can't. It's literally impossible. And that's why so many of us who are running ourselves into unbearable depletion also, somehow, absurdly, feel like failures—which seems ludicrous, right?! How is that possible with how much we actually do (and do well) on a daily basis? How is it possible that we see ourselves as failures with how much we pour into our kids and our careers and our relationships every minute we're awake?

## Make a Different List

I think I figured it out though. We're making the wrong lists. When I was a mom to a four-year-old, a two-year-old, and a newborn, I was making the wrong lists. As a mom to teens and a tween, I've been making the wrong lists. At the end of the day, when we look back at what we didn't get done since whatever ungodly hour we woke up, we're making the wrong lists.

Here's what I mean. How often do you look back at your day, weekend, week, month, or year, and list all the things you didn't do? Now, how about this: how often do you list the things you DID do?

For example (and I expand on this in Chapter 12), I try to drink 100 oz. of water a day. Every single day, I embark upon this challenge. And every single day, I fail. Mostly because I'm so damn busy chauffeuring around three kids without time to stop and pee and also because they were all 9 lbs. at birth so my bladder is teetering on the brink of malfunction most of the day.

I also try to have a clean house. Again, I have never once succeeded at this endeavor. I live with four other humans and an 80-lb. dog. Not one of these living creatures really seems too worried about the level of cleanliness in our home, which leads to lots of challenges (and surprises) like socks stuffed in the couch cushions, dirty drink cups on every single table, counter, and flat surface we own, and tufts of dog hair floating by like it's Oklahoma in 1935. That means, some days, yeah, I call it in and say, "*Welp, this house looks like the Johnson family lives here.*" Because we do. And that's that.

I also try to work out every day.

And volunteer at my kids' school.

And practice self-care.

And read more books. (Remember my "someday" dream?!)

And you can see the pattern here ... fail, fail, fail, and fail.

I work out ... sometimes.

I volunteer ... on occasion.

Self-care, book reading—yes they happen, but never as often as I hope to or plan for.

But one day I had an epiphany—one of those life-changing realizations. I'd had one of those badass Joe Efficient days (or should I say *Josephine* Efficient)—anyway, you know the ones. You work out. You eat healthy. You deep clean your kitchen. You tackle a big project for your job. You just feel truly accomplished as you look back on your day. And then the self-doubt creeps in, as you realize all the things on that "other" list you didn't achieve. On this particular day, I'd make a healthy meal for my kids—with a green vegetable! AND THEY ATE IT. I exercised. I drank buckets of water (still probably not 100 oz. but whatever). I cleaned. I organized. I was an Energizer bunny, and I felt so damn good.

Until I realized that I'd ignored my kids all day long. Because the only way to be super productive when pulling the to-do tasks out of one bucket is to ignore another bucket. And almost as quickly as I'd felt proud of myself, the air began to deflate out of my accomplishment balloon and the old narrative crept into my head: "*You're a failure.*"

"*No*," I said to myself. "*Fuck no.*" This time, I didn't let those negative intrusive thoughts win. My kids ate a damn vegetable! How could I possibly feel like a failure? I vowed from that day on that for every list I was to make about all the things I didn't get done, I'd make an equally long list of what I did accomplish, and I'd write that one in bigger, brighter font in my mind. On sparkly paper. Scented, even, like Elle Woods would. Because that's the kind of list we need to show ourselves.

Here's the truth. Some days, I'm Super Fun Mom and we play board games, go on walks together, watch a marathon of Marvel movies, and eat too much sugar. On those days, I don't clean or work out or pay bills or do 186 things that were on my list. But how can I look at those days as failures? Other days, my kids are left to entertain themselves while I work several hours on the computer writing articles, then scrub the kitchen floor, and clean out the coat closet. Are those days failures? Hell no.

But never—not one single day—will I ever cross off every item on my "mom/default-parent/wife/writer" to-do list. Ever. It's impossible. So, I can choose to spend the rest of my days looking at myself as a failure when I only achieve a few. Or I can say, "Look at me being awesome, getting shit done" as I give 100 percent.

And I'm telling you, if you put that second list at top billing in your mind, your mental health will feel a boost. You will realize how much you're succeeding, not failing. That old narrative of "*I didn't get everything done today*" is replaced by "*I didn't do it all, but I did a few things pretty damn well, which makes me a fucking rockstar.*"

## Notes on Chapter 3

*Can we really change our mindsets about "doing it all?" Yep? And we need to as we enter this next chapter in our lives.*

Because here's the truth: as we think about what we're going to be when the kids grow up, those same old toxic narratives are going to creep back in about how we can "have it all." (Society has made sure they're reeeeeeally embedded deep within us.) And even though we might not have little ones under our feet anymore while we cook mac and cheese and spread peanut butter and jelly on bread before cutting the crusts off, we're still moms. We'll still have endless obligations. Our young adult kids will need our help with their taxes and figuring out what to do when their car breaks down or the roof at their apartment is leaking. And for many of us in the sandwich generation, our parents will need us more and more too in the coming years.

That day my kids ate broccoli and I worked out and drank water and cleaned my house and was Josephine Efficient (but ignored my kids all day) will look like a lot of days in the future, even if my kids are (hopefully) eating green veggies in their own houses. I'll never not have a list and you'll never not have a list. You'll never be done battling the voices in your head that say you're not good enough because you didn't get it all done.

So, as you figure out what's next for you, start practicing these four things:

1. Make your list—the right one. The one that reminds you how successful your day was.
2. Tell yourself this: "You're doing a good job." Write it on a Post-it and stick it to your mirror.
3. Accept and make peace with the truth that you can't do it all. Remind yourself that no one else can either. Keep saying that to yourself—this is a lie we've been told and it's unachievable. You're a success.
4. Re-read your list.

Also, read this tweet:

> **21stcenturysahm**
>
> The one common thing among every mom I know — regardless of race or ethnicity or religion or political party or where you live or how old you are or how many kids you have is this: every mom I know works tirelessly for her kids every single day. Never stops. Carries her kids' joy, pain, successes, failures & everything in between. Never gives up.
>
> And not one gives herself the credit she deserves. Not one says out loud "I'm doing a good job." But you are. We all are. Why can't we see it?

# Chapter 4

# When Mothers Are Ghosts

"*Sometimes I feel like a ghost. Like they don't even see me.*" My sister said this to me once about motherhood and how she feels like her work goes unnoticed. I thought it was so profound and accurately depicted how so many of us feel as we carry the invisible load for our loved ones. An invisible load of work that, if we don't do it, would cause our entire family's house of cards to tumble and fall.

It's the sports uniforms that get magically cleaned and hung up, ready for the next game.

It's the food that just appears in the fridge and the snacks that are always in the pantry, ready for the kids and their friends to grab before retreating back to their rooms or the basement to resume their video games.

It's the activities that the children are all of a sudden registered for. The endless forms—poof—are filled out. So they were five pages long and took 90 minutes out of the mother's day to complete. Who else knows the pediatrician's name, number, address, insurance info, and who to put down for emergency contacts?

*The emails sent to the teachers. The permission slips signed. The report cards checked. The parent-teacher conferences attended, even if they're in the middle of the day. She'll make it work.*

*The well visit appointments made for the pediatrician. And the dentist. And the orthodontist. And the dermatologist.*

*The new shoes bought because their feet keep growing.*

*The back to school supplies purchased—every glue stick, no. 2 pencil, and loose-leaf notebook on the list.*

*The first day outfits picked out and haircuts done and pictures taken even though they whined and you were rushed, but now the memories are forever preserved.*

*It's the "Oh no! I forgot to buy a ticket for the dance!" panic. Don't worry, Mom already got it for you. (She did it the day she took you shopping for the dress. And the shoes. And the jewelry. She didn't forget.)*

*It's the running to the store for last minute art project supplies and a birthday gift—the party is tomorrow! "Sorry, Mom, didn't I mention it?"*

*It's the "Mom, can you help me study because I'm stressed about this test (but also don't nag me about my grade. Ugh, I can handle it, Mom.)"*

She's always there—Mom. She's in the background, a specter, an apparition who floats in and out, delicately navigating that space between being needed but making sure to not hover too much.

Much of her work is invisible, and no one even gives it much thought. More bread appears on the counter so everyone can have sandwiches. New socks appear in drawers as old ones have holes in the toe. Fresh toothbrushes are suddenly on the bathroom sink (old ones tossed in the trash).

To everyone else, these things just happen. And because oftentimes her work goes unappreciated and unnoticed, she might feel like an apparition no one sees.

But the truth is, the ghost in the background is the keeper of all the keys. She knows how this one doesn't like mayonnaise on his sandwiches, and that one has an algebra test tomorrow that's really stressing her out.

She knows which kid is doing well with friendships right now and which one is feeling left out.

She senses when they are on the cusp of change, quietly supporting the shift from "dark makeup Emo-girl" to "crop-top wearing Swiftie" that happens overnight. She sees it happening before it even happens and is ready in the wings to clean out the old to make room for the new so that her child feels seen and validated and loved, no matter what phase she's in.

She knows when they need to be picked up off the floor and when they feel on top of the world and just need her to look up with pride, ready to hold the trophy so they can go celebrate with friends. She's the reason they were even there to win the trophy in the first place. She was the ride to and from every practice, she was the sign-up captain, she knew the game schedule, and she was the one who made sure the fridge was stocked with first and second dinners all week long.

She's the puppet-master, pulling all the strings. Some call her a "control freak" but really, she just knows that if one bolt on that Ferris wheel comes loose (see Chapter 6)—one misstep, one forgotten task, one miscue on the family calendar—that the whole structure can come crashing down. And that she, the mother, will be the one to put it all back together.

No one understands that even as she sleeps, the machine keeps whirring. Like a ghost, she never rests.

It's why she forgets to take care of herself. (*Ghosts don't need anything to exist.*)

It's why she walked away from her career. (*Ghosts are invisible, easy to miss.*)

She feels pride and gratitude for all of it. But she also feels like a ghost and sometimes wonders if anyone sees her at all.

---

## Notes on Chapter 4

*We're not ghosts. We're real, we're here, and we are so necessary that if we did actually disappear, everything would crumble and fall. So, here are two things you can do when you feel like a ghost that will help you remember you're not:*

1. **Recognize that you are a whole, real person with needs.**

    You can (and should) assert yourself to your family when you don't feel seen or appreciated. But in the end, it might be on you to put color back on the picture of Mom. You might need to outline your silhouette in the family portrait yourself. But how? By doing something entirely for you. Breathe life back into yourself by doing something that's not about them, but instead, about you. Go to a coffee shop for the day and read a book. Take a girls' weekend trip. Go hiking for the day. Disappear—for real—for a hot minute and your absence will be felt immediately. A little reminder for your family of all you do (which they'll notice when you don't do it) is an effective way to ensure that you're noticed when you return! (And while you're gone, spoiling yourself a little bit is just an added bonus.)

2. **Write down your actual name (not "Mom") and think about who she is.**

    When motherhood cloaks us in invisibility, we need to remember that we are also someone else. I'm a mom but I'm also Karen Johnson, writer. Karen Johnson, former teacher. Karen Johnson, wife, daughter, sister, friend. Karen Johnson, lover of books, glasses of wine with girlfriends, and traveling the world.

    When you feel like a ghost, remember the whole other part of you. She's still there. Bring her back to the surface. Write out your name and a list of who that person is. Then go do something with her. Right now, Karen Johnson, writer, is at a coffee shop on a Saturday writing this chapter, and she's full of life. What do you want to do? What do you want to be?

# Chapter 5

# How Much Are SAHMs Actually Worth?

I talk to my children a lot about self-worth. I want them to know that they are worth more than their GPA, more than a number on a scale, more than the tag on their clothing. They are worth more than the number of goals they score or how well they perform on a standardized test or how many kids from the popular group message them on Snapchat.

Where, then, does worth come from? A person's worth is determined by what they contribute to society. How they impact the greater good. What they put out into the space around them. Are they kind? Compassionate? Do they have a strong worth ethic? Are they honest?

And this conversation is important because, inevitably, life will push our children down and they will at some point question their value in this world. And it's our job as parents to ensure that the foundation is in place—that the source of their self-worth is there—so they land on solid footing.

But what about us moms? What about when we question our worth and value? How do we remind ourselves of just how vital we are to everyone and everything around us?

## The Cost to Replace a Mother

Years ago, my husband and I were having one of those awkward and terrifying but very necessary adult conversations about death, wills, and life insurance. And that meant we had to talk money—namely, what we were each "worth" if we suddenly turned to dust.

Talking about his "value" or "worth" when it comes to life insurance was pretty easy (I mean, not "easy" because we're talking about him *dying*, but you know what I mean). In our family, and in lots of families with a stay-at-home parent, I might steer the ship, but he pays for it. All five of us are well aware that we have a home, food, heat and electricity, and fun stuff like travel hockey and family vacations because of Dad's paycheck (not Mom's). So yeah, when we talked over life insurance policies, we decided pretty quickly that he needed a big one.

And honestly, I thought that was it.

Until he asked, *"What about you?"*

Ummm ... me? The former teacher turned SAHM turned writer who hasn't had a steady income in 15 years and sometimes goes months making zilch?

*"Why would I have a life insurance policy?"* I asked, laughing.

And that's when he explained my worth in a way I hadn't seen it before. That even though I don't bring much money into the household, I'm actually a very valuable (very expensive) asset.

*"Do you know what I'd have to do if something happened to you? The number of people I'd have to hire? We're absolutely getting a life insurance policy for you and a big one,"* he said.

And he was right. He works long hours and travels sometimes for work. We'd need a nanny 24/7. A driver. A homework helper. A grocery getter.

We'd need someone to remember about signups for camp and baseball tryouts and horseback riding lessons. Someone to make sure we had solid black clothes and shoes that fit for theater for one kid and sharpened ice skates and a helmet that fit for another. Someone who had reminders set for the trumpet lessons and dermatology appointments and all the other lessons and appointments in between (and the means and time to get the kids to all of them). Someone who could read a kid's temperature with the back of their hand and assess in real time whether they needed to see a doctor or just wait it out. (And who could immediately clear their schedule to tend to whatever sickness was now in the house.)

And we'd definitely, 100%, need a cleaning service.

It's not that my husband isn't willing to do these things—it's that it wouldn't cross his mind to check on tennis registration or make sure everyone has clean underwear or run a vacuum in the living room. And even if I was no longer here, even if he did think of it, he wouldn't have time because of how many hours per week he works.

I realized in that conversation that I wear many hats: chef, chauffeur, nurse, house cleaner, paperwork filler-outer, registrar, personal assistant, family calendar manager extraordinaire…. It would really take a village to do everything I do. And how much does a village cost? A lot, I'd imagine.

SAHMs, we need to change how we define our worth and value, so that we don't feel like ghosts (see Chapter 4). Our labor might be unpaid, but look at how valuable it is. Imagine your household if you went poof—and disappeared. Imagine the team that would have to be brought in to do all of your jobs. Imagine the expense of you—the sheer cost of what it would take.

Our value as SAHMs is often diminished because our labor is free and because so many of us never actually feel truly successful. We can't ever get everything done, and we feel perpetually exhausted, overwhelmed, and defeated. But when our husbands and partners come home looking exhausted, overwhelmed, and defeated, at least there's a paycheck tied to all of it.

But not for us.

And yes, we might have loved ones try to build us up and say things like, "But YOUR job is the MOST important of all! You keep the kids safe every day!" And while, yes, that's true, it doesn't often *feel* like the most important of all. It often feels lonely and empty and insignificant.

## Don't Let Some Idiot at a Wedding Diminish Your Worth

Here's the truth: even though we never stop working all day long, it can be hard to feel valuable when society says that we're not. A long time ago, when the big kids were babies and I was drowning in SAHM overwhelm, we attended a wedding for college friends. It was a big deal for me, and every single insecurity I was feeling came pouring out. The bride was younger than I was and I had convinced myself that all the women were going to be cute and trendy in their pre-kids selves. I didn't even own a dress that fit—what did people wear to weddings anymore? What did *breastfeeding moms* wear to weddings?!

But I bought a dress, did my hair and makeup, and hit the party, ready to let loose a little. And that's when it happened. At a table full of young professionals, someone asked me that dreaded question: "*What do you do?*"

"*I'm a former teacher, but now I'm a stay-at-home mom,*" I answered.

And what he said in response is forever seared into my brain. That man literally said to me, "*I'd love to be a stay-at-home dad so I could sit on the couch all day and watch TV.*"

Yup, he actually said that. And it hurt. My husband immediately jumped to my defense as I sat there, seething with anger. Even that idiot's wife called him out on making such an asinine comment.

At that time in my life, I was the sole caregiver most days from morning until night, keeping a four-year-old, two-year-old, and a breastfeeding baby alive, but I allowed that dingbat to cut right through me with his ignorant statement. And yes, while I was doing the most important work in the world: raising contributing members of society and future grown adults who would never insult another person by making rude comments at a damn wedding, I was also saving my family a shit-ton of money.

Because guess what?

What that buffoon probably didn't know (or else he'd have said something kinder and more respectful to me) is that the average SAHM, if she earned an income for everything she does, is worth $186,000 a year.[1]

That's because when you consider the actual cost of raising a child, you realize quickly how valuable a SAHM really is. For example, check out these jaw-dropping stats (courtesy of care.com):

- The average weekly nanny cost is $766.
- The average weekly daycare cost is $321.
- The average weekly family care center cost is $230.
- And the average weekly babysitter cost is $192.

Also, how about cleaning services? That's going to cost you around $20 an hour.

What about formula? As a mom who exclusively breastfed, I fed my babies for FREE, saving us, according to smartasset.com, between $800 and $3,000 per year.[2] And multiply that times three because I did it three times!

Seeing these numbers, imagine the cost of hiring a person to meal plan, grocery shop or order groceries, cook, do laundry, schedule doctor's appointments, dentist appointments, haircuts, buy new clothes, help with homework after school, drive all the kids to their various activities, etc., etc., etc.

So yeah, when I actually thought about it, I realized I am worth A LOT. A freaking fortune, in fact. And replacing me would require some serious wo(man)power. So to that loser wedding

---

[1] https://www.salary.com/articles/how-much-is-a-mom-really-worth-the-amount-may-surprise-you.
[2] https://smartasset.com/financial-advisor/the-cost-of-baby-formula.

guest at my table, *I do a hell of a lot more than sit on the couch and watch TV all day.*

Moms, you're worth much more than you realize. (And yes, you need life insurance.)

---

## Notes on Chapter 5

*Moms, remember these numbers and statistics when:*

1. **You start thinking about what's next for you and you feel guilty about the expense.**

    Want to go back to school or launch into a new career? Need to buy books or pay tuition or invest in your own business or buy a new wardrobe? Well, if you've been a SAHM for a couple decades like I have, look at how much money you have saved and don't feel guilty for a damn second.

2. **Some donkey at a wedding makes one of those idiotic "What do you do all day?" comments.**

    Ummm ... working multiple full-time jobs and keeping small humans alive, Chad. What do YOU do?

3. **You feel invisible or unappreciated.**

    Your family would not be able to afford to replace you. You are literally PRICELESS.

## Chapter 6

# The Default Parenting Ferris Wheel

When you became a mom, did you know you were also signing up to work a carnival ride? I sure didn't. But it's true, and only default parents carrying the mental load (most commonly mothers) understand the giant default parenting Ferris wheel that never stops moving, and how even one loose bolt can bring the whole thing to a screeching halt.

And knowing how fragile the wheel is (and how the entire family relies on us to keep it spinning), it's not surprising when we turn into fire-breathing dragons and try to burn the entire fair down as we hear seemingly simple one-fits-all solutions like *"Mom needs to delegate jobs to other people!"* or *"Stop doing everything for your kids! They need to learn consequences!"*

We know you mean well with these suggestions, and we 100 percent agree that kids SHOULD learn consequences and we'd LOVE to have help with the mental load.

However.

The thing is, it's not a super stable wheel—it's a little rickety and any strong wind can come along and knock it over. And when I say "strong wind," I mean things like the stomach flu. Or lice. Or even a "slight breeze" like the kids missing the bus that morning or forgetting their lunch at home.

And moms who are running the wheel know this balancing act and how vital it is that all of their 27 proverbial limbs (I think that's how many we have, give or take a few) continue to hold up all of the wheel's constantly moving parts. That's why we "*do too much for our kids*" and don't always "*just let them learn consequences!*" Because, yes, it is my child's responsibility to bring his lunch to school and if he forgets, "*Oh well! He'll be hungry for the day and learn his lesson!*" right? Except my child has food allergies and often can't eat school lunch and then probably has practice after school, so he'll be hungry, won't feel well, and then he'll be an emotional train wreck for the rest of the night.

And do you know who will be picking up the "nuts and bolts" that fell off that day (i.e. the inevitable hangry meltdown he'll have at 9 p.m.)? You guessed it—Mom.

Also, Carnival Ferris Wheel Default Parent Mental Load Carrying Moms (that's our full and complete title: CFWDPMLCM for short) know why it's so infuriating when we're told to just "delegate" roles off our mental checklist. For example, "*Register child for camp.*" That's an easy one to pass off, right? Wrong. Veteran moms know that camps fill up in about 11.5 seconds, which means this one is high level. And if you miss it and don't snag a spot, guess who is now consoling a disappointed child and who *also is now responsible for figuring out what to do with said child who was supposed to be at camp this summer*?! Yeah, you're looking at her. She might as well just register the kid herself.

This is why we do it all and why we are sometimes angry that we're doing it all.

*Brush your teeth!* Why? Because if you get a cavity, guess who has to take time off to take you to the dentist? Mom.

*Eat a vegetable.* Why? Because if you get sick due to a diet that's nothing but processed garbage, you'll never poop, you won't be able to focus in school, your grades will suffer, you won't play well, the coach will sit you, you'll be an emotional honey badger, and guess who will feel the fallout the most? Mom.

(Also, guess who society judges when the world sees you eating fruit snacks and chugging a Coke? Mom. And to be honest (tbh), we don't need the side-eye. We question ourselves enough.)

*Bring down your laundry.* Why? Because the washing machine is currently empty, you need a clean uniform for tomorrow, and if we don't do it now, we'll all forget and it won't be ready in the morning. Who is always thinking 14 steps ahead? Mom.

*Wash the dishes.* Why? Because do you know who has a permanent footprint the shape of her feet in front of the sink and deserves a damn break? Mom. But also, who knows full well that tomorrow morning when you're scarfing down a bowl of cereal before school that there will be no cleans spoons unless we run the dishwasher tonight? MOM KNOWS.

*Do your homework.* Why? So you can graduate and someday give Mom a rest from running this circus.

All we ask is that the other people in our lives do their part, too, to keep the wheel moving. If we ask you to put your shoes away, just do it. Why? So you'll know where they are when we're rushing out the door tomorrow and we won't be late for an activity we've already signed you up and paid for.

Because even something as simple as size six boys' sneakers that have gone missing is enough to jolt one screw out of place. And then the wheel comes to a screeching halt and bit by bit, other pieces begin to come off. But because we're incredibly good at keeping the wheel going, we already anticipated this bolt coming loose—even when no one else did. And that's why we just need you to put your freaking shoes away where they go so the wheel can keep turning and Mom can continue to meet everyone's needs.

Listen, no one told us we'd be carnival workers when we signed up for motherhood, but here we are. Please just bring us a funnel cake and maybe fold the damn towels. We got shit to do and this ride never stops moving.

## Notes on Chapter 6

*Hot tip on how to make sure the wheel never stops turning:*
You can't. (I know, not the answer you were hoping for.)
Here's the hard truth: The ride's going to break down at some point. It just is. I know, I know, we are doing everything! How is it still not enough? Because life gets life-y and sometimes we simply run out of energy to keep it going. So what then? What do we do when a bolt comes loose?

We accept it.

That's it.

I've worked on this one a lot in therapy. My dear savior therapist who is one of my very favorite humans (read more about her in Chapter 13) tells me this, which I hate hearing: Sometimes when you have all the balls in the air, one drops. It just does. And you have to accept it.

When she first told me this, I had a visceral reaction and I'm pretty sure I responded with a resounding "NOOOOOO" and shook my head in denial. But eventually I realized she was right. We have to accept this truth, let ourselves drop a ball now and then, and give ourselves grace even when it's hard (see Chapter 29: "We Can Do Hard Things").

Do I wish I had a more novel response and a solution so that we could all keep our carnival Ferris wheels continuously turning? Of course. But everything breaks at some point—including Mom.

Listen, when your wheel breaks down because your kid puked all over their bed or you forgot about an appointment or the car died on the side of the road and you see your dilapidated Ferris wheel turned over on its side, remember this: You'll get it back up and running. It's just in for repairs, getting a little tune-up, maybe some fresh bolts and screws, a shot or two of oil in the hinges, and will be shiny and ready to spin again. You're doing a good job, even when the wheels come off.

Also, maybe it's time for Mom to get a tune-up, too. Why don't you sneak in a mani-pedi (or a nap!) while it's in the shop?

## Chapter 7

# That Day I Hiked 14 Miles and Braced for a Hip Replacement (But Also Realized Something about Me as a Mom)

After a decade and a half of parenting and nearly two full decades of marriage, we've learned that in order to truly talk and have a real, meaningful conversation about, well, anything other than "*What's for dinner*" or "*Did anyone feed the dog?*" my husband and I have to escape. We have to drive away from the house, the children, the needy dog, the turtles who fight (see Chapter 23 about the hot mess that is our pet situation), and any other distraction that is likely to interrupt us in 45-second intervals.

And since we're not old but not young anymore, we also enjoy embarking on the occasional physical challenge, mostly because exercise is good for us, but also just to prove to ourselves and to each other that we still got it! We can still kayak down a river or go for a short run or hike to the top of a (small) mountain, right?

Last fall, we were able to escape for a "day date" so we decided to enjoy the last of the foliage season and complete an all-day hike. It ended up being a 14-miler, and although we were proud of ourselves, lots of things hurt afterwards as well (namely our knees and hip joints, but hey! We did it! So what if we needed to ice our muscles and go to bed early! #worthit, right?)

We left the house at 7 a.m. and were back home by dinner. It was a beautiful hiking day—warm enough to just wear a sweatshirt, cool enough to not be too sweaty when we hit a pub afterwards for a couple beers and some greasy food.

And we covered A LOT of ground (literally—14 miles is 14 miles, folks) but also with all the things we talked about. Dream vacations, possible house renovations, the kids' futures, our futures.

It was the perfect day to spend time together, just the two of us.

Except my phone dinged 12 times. TWELVE. On a day that I was "escaping" and "getting away" from all of my household manager roles.

And guess how many times my husband's phone went off?

0. As in ZE. RO.

"Mom, can I go to _____'s [insert friend's name] house?"

"Mom, can _____ [insert friend's name] come over?"

"Mom, do you know where my gray hoodie is?"

"Mom, _____ [insert sibling's name] ate the last bagel. What else is there for breakfast?!"

"Mom, isn't it _____'s [insert sibling's name] turn to walk the dog?"

"Mom, what time is practice tonight?"

"Mom, what time is practice tomorrow night?"

And the real kicker is that I had spent hours organizing their lives so that we *could* get away for a day. I'd lined up Grandma to take one to theater rehearsal and another to a friend's house. I made sure there was enough food to last A DAY (although—gasp!—there may have been a bagel shortage). I left a list of chores that, if done properly, should have consumed their time enough where there really wasn't any question of who was in charge of what, nor was there time for sibling arguing.

And yet.

## Why My Husband Really Can't Win (Sorry, Honey)

But here's the truth—a truth that often makes my husband's head spin off in frustration. As a default parent mom, I don't want the texts to go to anyone else. If the kids had bugged him all day, I'd be looking over his shoulder, asking "*What does she want? What is he eating for lunch? Who is walking the dog? Who is going to what friend's house? How are they getting there? Who else is going over there because that one friend is being mean lately and I'm not sure she'd want to go if the other girl is going. ... What time will they be home? Did they clean their room first?*"

I don't know how to shut it off or truly escape, but tbh, I'm not sure I want to.

I talk a lot about the exhaustion and overwhelm of default parenting, and I'll continue to do so because we need to normalize all parents sharing the mental load and give grace to moms trying to juggle it all.

However.

I'm also a big old hypocrite because if anyone tried to pry it all away from me—my job as keeper of the family calendar and the household manager role and all the knowledge about the kids' lives and friendship circles and who has what science test tomorrow and who got teased at recess last week—well, I'd hold onto all of it with a death grip. This much I know.

Is it because I've done it all and carried it all for 16 years that there is no other option in my brain? Is it because I believe wholeheartedly that I am the best person in my household, the most equipped, the best at multitasking, and, frankly, the one who *should* be in charge of the default parenting Ferris wheel because, as this book has referenced 9,831 times, I don't have a full-time career?

Or is it because my identity is so wrapped up in motherhood and SAHM-life that the thought of relinquishing any control at all rips the ground out from under me—because who would I be if I wasn't the keeper of all the keys?

All of these reasons are why when I *do* get away for a day, or even a weekend, I write lists upon lists of instructions, information, and schedules. Why I check in so much and why my phone is never, ever off and why, if I'm brave enough to take my 40-something self on a 14-mile hike one beautiful fall day, that my phone dings 12 times and I answer every single time.

I described the experience of default parenting as running a rickety Ferris wheel in Chapter 6. We have to keep the wheel moving and one lost shoe or slight fever or missed appointment can derail the whole thing. That's why it's not surprising that moms like me have extreme anxiety about a bolt coming loose and the whole wheel crashing to the ground if we're gone for a day. Because we all know who will be crawling around, on her hands and knees, scrambling to pick up the pieces so she can reassemble the wheel and get it back up and running when she gets home. And her name is Mom.

Also, many of us have been battling unrealistic perfectionism since we were like seven, so there's that, too. (I delve into that mess in Chapter 15.) Coming home to the household being in a complete disarray means that "taking a break" or "getting away" is really a punishment for us life-long perfectionists. It's often just easier to continue to micromanage it all from afar. Even if we're poolside in Vegas with our college besties, we might still pick up when the kids call asking where their cleats are. "*They're in the closet under the stairs,*" we'll respond, then go back to sipping our margaritas and catching up with old friends.

So, no, we can't just "hand off" the mental load or "take a break" and "get away for the day" when we are the default parent 1,000 percent of the time.

But also, we sort of don't want to, and that means that our partners can't actually win here. Sorry, honey. Thanks for your help. We appreciate you.

### Insert Gratitude Here

And also, here's another layer: You might have a partner like mine who sometimes gets a little envious of my life, just as I do of his.

We recently had a heavy, but important conversation about this. I was carrying all of the kids' proverbial "stuff" and he was at a big meeting in another country, feeling important in his thriving career. As I lamented that I was jealous of his fancy dinners while we ate leftovers at home, his response was important for me to hear.

*"But you're there. You know everything. You don't miss any of it. I hear about big stuff that they are going through sometimes days later. I know you envy what I have and what I get to do, but I envy what you have, too."*

It was really important for me to hear his perspective because I hadn't seen it that way before.

Maybe you're frustrated that your partner won't help. Or maybe your partner will but you don't know how to accept help. Or maybe you desperately want to keep all of it—the whole wheel, all the keys, all the knowledge, because you're terrified of what or who you'll be in the void—and you just want to be seen and appreciated.

All of those feelings are valid.

But particularly for anyone out there feeling jealousy or resentment, I'll tell you that for me, the best shield to fend off that negativity is gratitude. Whether it's resentment of your partner, jealousy of a friend, neighbor, family member who seems to have it all, or the toxicity of comparing yourself to other moms who seem to have their shit together while you're firmly seated on the hot mess express, practicing gratitude can be very effective at blocking out a lot of those damaging thoughts.

In this instance, it was helpful to hear my husband's words and feel grateful that, yes, I have been there for everything. I know all the things and I carry all of their "stuff." I am on the inside track, whether that's where I want to be 100 percent of the time or whether I'd occasionally like a mental break to step off for a hot second, but it's true. Default parenting and carrying the mental load is a freaking lot and there is no escape. Ever. But it's also a beautiful blessing and I know that someday I won't need so many keys. Someday, that big old rickety Ferris wheel will stop turning. Someday, if those old hips will let me, I'll go hiking and not receive 12 texts because my kids will have stepped off at some point and gone on to live their own lives.

And I'll be grateful that I was there for every minute of the ride.

## Notes on Chapter 7

*Three reasons why gratitude helps with the overwhelm of motherhood:*
We've been climbed on, needed, had our boobs gnawed on, and had our side of the bed stolen for decades. It's all we've known, which means giving any of it up feels like our skin is being ripped off. And yet, we're desperate for another identity at the same time. Here's how actively practicing gratitude helps me work through feeling both of those things simultaneously:

**1. It improves my relationships.**

With my husband (as described above), but also, with my kids. When I'm in the car for the eleventh time in one day, I might be so damn tired of holding on to that steering wheel and driving out of my driveway AGAIN. But maybe this drive is when I get to hear what's going on with my 14-year-old daughter and her friend group. Or how my 16-year-old is feeling about his upcoming junior year's course load. Or that my youngest is actually a lot more stressed about middle school than he's been letting on.

I'm grateful and don't want anyone else in that driver's seat for those important conversations.

## 2. It reminds me of my purpose and value.

I am grateful I get to be there for everything. I am grateful that when my kids look back at their childhoods, they'll remember that I was always there, that they always saw me in the stands or always knew I was waiting to pick them up, wanting to hear how it all went, and ready to offer a celebratory "congrats!" or a comforting shoulder when it didn't go so well.

Feeling gratitude for all my jobs (and there are a lot!) helps with my feelings of invisibility in motherhood and helps me feel more valued on the days I feel like a ghost.

## 3. It helps with my mental health.

When I feel depressed or anxious about everything motherhood demands of me, gratitude helps me cope. That doesn't mean I stop asking for help or continue to take it all on if I'm burnt out. And it doesn't mean I abandon necessary self-care to cope with my mental health struggles (see Chapter 13). But it does mean I stop and think about how crucial I am to my household and how valuable it is that my kids know I'm always there, in person or a text away.

# Chapter 8

# "Hi, I'm Sweating!" (WTF Is Happening to My Body?)

I have a question and that question is this: What. Is. Happening? Why isn't there a giant neon blinking sign on the roadway of life as we stroll out of our 30s and enter our fourth decade that reads:

- *"WARNING! PREPARE TO EITHER BE FREEZING OR SWEATING EVERY MINUTE OF EVERY DAY NOW!*
- *ALSO, YOU'RE GOING TO GAIN A BUNCH OF RANDOM, UNEXPECTED WEIGHT AND HAVE NO IDEA WHAT YOUR CLOTHING SIZE IS EVER.*
- *AND FINALLY, YOU DON'T SLEEP ANYMORE.*
- *GODSPEED."*

And to make it all worse, the diet and beauty industries know exactly what they're doing, tapping into alllllll of our insecurities.

*"Buy this cream! Take this pill! Follow this diet! Look younger! Be skinnier! Spend all your money trying to prevent aging even though that's a losing battle and you can't stop it! Also for some infuriating reason, men are totally allowed to age, but we're not—don't get mad about it though because angry, scowling faces look old! Just buy more products and smile!"*

Also, while perimenopause hits like a Mack truck, (*You get your period! No you don't! Yes you do! You might be pregnant at 44! Or you're a menopausal grandmother! Hahahaha, how fun is this?*) you're also starting to worry about breast cancer. *"Check your boobs!"* we're told, on top of everything else. And *"Take calcium supplements to keep those bones dense because osteoporosis is coming for you as well!"*

And then they'll tell us to practice self-care and wonder why we're crying into our sweat-covered pillows.

Honestly, it's a lot to process and a heads-up would have been nice.

Growing up, we knew about a few huge life-changing events: getting our period, having babies, and menopause (a special something reserved for Grandma). That was it. No one talked about perimenopause. We didn't know that was a thing.

We didn't know that because we have female reproductive organs, every single year after we turn eight would likely be consumed with drastic physical change that meant we didn't know what size pants we were, why our boobs hurt, or whether we were falling asleep walking because of hormones, pregnancy, or just the immense weight of the patriarchy.

WE NEED TO TALK ABOUT THIS SHIT MORE.

For me, the big changes started at around age 38. Prior to that, I'd always been around the same size throughout my adult life. Even after all the kids were born, my body eventually returned to its standard shape, weight, and clothing size. I had no reason to think it someday would drastically change, but oh how naive I was.

The weight came on fast and furious and by the time I hit my early 40s, it seemed like I had a totally different body than the one I'd lived in for the past 15 to 20 years.

Coupled with a new stubborn gray hair sprouting up every other day (why do they have to stick straight up?!), a completely irregular menstrual cycle, and unforeseen bouts of exhaustion that pretty much take my legs out from under me, it can be hard sometimes to feel, well, positive about the "me" looking back at me.

Especially when not only do my clothes consistently not fit year after year but also, in whatever I do manage to drag out of my closet and bravely wear out into the world, there's a 92 percent chance I've got pit stains and a bead of perspiration developing on my upper lip.

I mean, who doesn't love breaking out into a sweat in the middle of the damn winter when everyone around you is snuggled up in a warm, cozy sweater? I get hot and anxious just looking at wool now.

Recently, I did some volunteer work in my town (a perk of being a mostly job-less mom!) and was attending a happy hour event afterwards with my fellow volunteers. I knew I'd have wine and I knew I'd get hot (and not in a good way). I came prepared (not my first rodeo) and wore layers. But it was chilly out and still "wintery" where I live, so stripping down to a tee seemed, well, weird. I held out as long as I could, chatting with friends from around town, feeling moisture drip down my back as the wine sweats took over my perimenopausal body.

Finally, I couldn't take it anymore, and I ripped off my cardigan, fearing the worst. I'd probably already pitted out. So, as any normal not-socially-awkward person would do, I just started stating facts. As each new person approached me for a hello (or God forbid a sweaty hug), I greeted them by saying, *"Hi! I'm sweaty! I think I'm pitting out."* (See Chapter 25 about how I'm always awkward.)

My volunteer services have not been requested since.

Anyway, that's how I like to party these days. Who wants to join me on this pit-stained roller coaster?

## Doing Better for Our Girls

But here's the twist, girlfriends.

You know what's empowering through all the muck of gaining weight and discovering rogue grays and feeling my temperature soar when I'm trying to look cute at a happy hour event? This body is stronger than ever—it's true. I lift heavier weights than I lifted when I was in my 20s. I do advanced fitness routines I'd never have attempted two decades ago. And I have carried three nine-pound babies to term, pushed them out into the world, and then nursed and carried them around while growing the next one. I am very aware of just how incredibly strong I am today even though some parts are bigger (and warmer) or shaped differently than they were years ago.

Here's a fact I want you to hear and remember: That body you see in the mirror deserves kindness. That body deserves love. And despite (and perhaps because of) all its scars and cellulite and imperfections, that body of yours deserves respect. And so does mine.

Also, because life is tricky that way, guess who is standing alongside us moms in our 40s, listening as we criticize our fat rolls and wrinkles and gray hairs? Our girls. Given that the most common age for childbirth is late 20s and early 30s, that means as many of us hit the physical challenges of perimenopause, our daughters are hitting all the physical changes of adolescence. And when we say hateful things about our bodies, they are listening—as their bodies are changing too. If we want them to embrace their own strong legs and arms, if we want them to think their faces and tummies are beautiful, even as they grow and morph into something new, well, that starts with us.

Have you ever watched old footage of the 1990s and early 2000s, at the height of the "thin is in" movement of our youth? Have you ever heard the interviews and horrific questions celebrities were asked about their weight? Or come across old headlines about whatever pop star was suddenly branded as "bigger" or even "fat" but you look at her now and realize she was actually maybe just not prepubescent or starving? Now imagine our kids growing up in a society where that's not normal and that's not okay. A world where Bridget Jones isn't "chubby," where our daughters aren't guilted into burning off every single calorie and instead are told to just enjoy a damn cookie because who doesn't love cookies? Where feeling healthy, eating real meals, and looking at their strong bodies in the mirror is the goal, not feeling hungry and watching themselves shrink?

Let's not imagine it. Let's do it for them.

Because not only do I want my daughter to love herself now, but I want her to love herself when she's 44, too. Someday, she might sweat through her shirt at a social event, and I want her to know that it's fine. She's still awesome even if she sticks her head in the freezer for a hot minute.

Honestly, the thought of my kind, creative daughter hating what she sees in the mirror her entire life is enough to bring me to my knees and swear on everything I believe that I will do better for her.

And maybe, just maybe, that means that I don't have to hate what I see in the mirror, too. Because the thing is, this is the best it's going to be. The grays are going to keep coming. The skin is going to keep sagging. The bones and muscles will only weaken as I age and the wrinkles around my eyes and mouth will only multiply.

Therefore, I have a choice. Take care of what I have and learn to cherish this one body I was given or berate it at every turn for the rest of my days. Aging means I've lived a life and that's all I can ask for—and all I can ask for my daughter to have as well.

Stop being your own worst bully and say something kind to yourself today. You don't have to love every single thing (who loves sweaty pits and rogue chin hairs?!) but pick something about you to love right now, at this moment. You deserve it. And also, your beautiful daughter might be listening.

## Notes on Chapter 8

*Here's some (kind of) advice:*

Listen, I'm not an expert. Or a therapist. Or a doctor. I wish I had the magical answer to stop sweating profusely, but I don't. I guess carry extra deodorant and a backup shirt in your car (like I do!) Also, wear layers so you can hide your pits.

But more importantly, here are a couple of social media posts I've shared over the years (and remember, I'm also talking to myself here) that I want you to see and hear, too. Get used to unapologetically loving, appreciating, accepting, and valuing yourself. Practice it. Say it. Model it. Wear clothes that fit and make you feel beautiful and allow you to eat and drink and experience life. Toss anything that doesn't. You deserve the joy that comes with loving your own self. And your kids do, too.

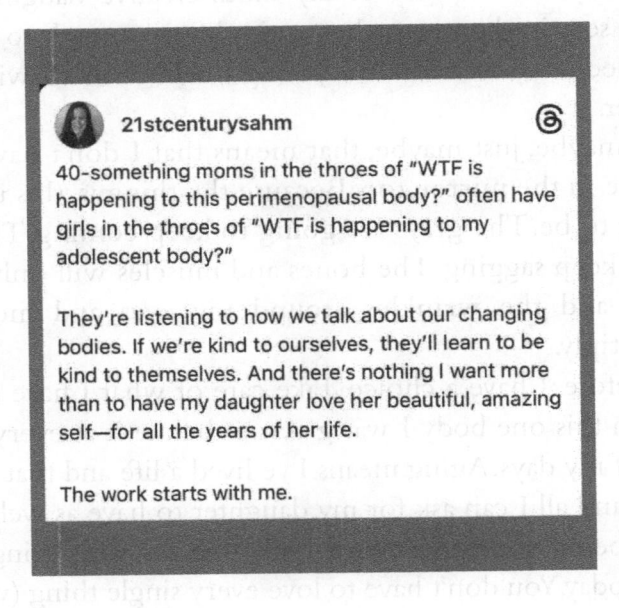

> **21stcenturysahm**
>
> 40-something moms in the throes of "WTF is happening to this perimenopausal body?" often have girls in the throes of "WTF is happening to my adolescent body?"
>
> They're listening to how we talk about our changing bodies. If we're kind to ourselves, they'll learn to be kind to themselves. And there's nothing I want more than to have my daughter love her beautiful, amazing self—for all the years of her life.
>
> The work starts with me.

## "Hi, I'm Sweating!" (WTF Is Happening to My Body?)

**21stcenturysahm** — now

Hey perimenopausal women whose bodies are changing drastically:

Remember that the diet industry 1000% relies on us hating ourselves. We can't let them win. We're in this together. Also, you're strong & amazing. Write that on a post it today & stick it to your mirror.

> In case you needed a reminder, here it is: The body you woke up in TODAY is a beach body. And a pool body. And a lake body. And a body deserving of any and all activities the summer might offer you. So is the body you'll wake up in tomorrow. And the one you'll wake up in come July.
>
> — The 21st Century SAHM
>
> So go live your life, enjoy the summer, go swimming if you want to, wear shorts if you want to, drink a beer and eat fried cheese if you want to. Laugh really loud, blast 90s music, take a million selfies, do what makes you happy. You deserve to feel joy, out in the world, in the body you have right now.

# Chapter 9

# On Aging and Beauty Culture (So, I Guess I Have a Turkey Neck Now...? Whatever)

One super fun physical surprise I've noticed as my 30s drifted off into the sunset and I careened toward I guess, "middle age" (which, btw, sounds like we should be using chamber pots as we avoid the Bubonic Plague) is that on several parts of my body, my skin appears to be ... looser.

And like so many other changes on the perimenopausal train that we're forced to board whether we want to or not, I did not see this one coming.

But it's happening. My skin is losing some of its elasticity and one of those body parts that's really wanting to give up, it seems, is my neck. So, there it is. A turkey neck. File it right under "*moles, frown lines, and random creepy eyelid wrinkles*" as yet another strange, but seemingly unavoidable sign that, yes, I am, in fact, getting older.

*"But it is avoidable!"* the beauty industry will tell us. *"You just need to spend your money on this $300 organic sheepskin collagen-filled tea tree oil neck mask! It will firm your neck skin right up (or not ... probably not ... we don't really know except we're going to tell you that it's 100 percent guaranteed knowing full well that if it doesn't work you're not going to actually go through the time and effort to contact our customer service and tell them that your damn stubborn neck skin is still fighting the good fight and just REFUSES to firm up so you'd like your 'Six easy installments of $50' back please) so order today! No one has to actually accept that they are aging! Don't spend your money on making memories, drinking delicious wine with your spouse, and eating ice cream with your kids by the beach! You'll be miserable hearing your children's laughter and seeing them splash in the waves if your loose neck skin is flapping in the wind."*

And it's not just the neck. Apparently, arms in our 30s do NOT look like arms in our 40s (at least not for me). Despite working out as hard (harder, actually) than I did years ago and being physically stronger than I've ever been, the skin elasticity plague has got me there, too. Right around 40, my arms just started looking different. And again, I didn't see it coming, and again, I had to decide if I'm going to:

1. Throw myself into some surgical arm-skin skin firming program (or, at the very least, buy absurdly expensive *"arm skin tightening cream"*—probably made by the neck skin mask people)
Or
2. Just accept that I'm 44, and my arms are 44. Just like my neck. This means accepting that I am aging, and that as I get older, my skin has a harder time fighting gravity. It means saying *"Whatever,"* cracking a beer, and sitting by the pool with my loose old neck and arms swinging in the breeze.

Choosing option two was pretty easy for me, mostly because I don't spend money on beauty products pretty much ever. I never have. I don't even dye my hair but, rather, have decided to let the grays creep in without a fight. So, it's not a huge leap for me to say "*Hell no*" when I see the price tag on "*skin-firming*" or "*anti-aging*" creams, lotions, masks, serums, gels, or crystals from the bottom of the Adriatic Sea. I'm just not doing it—turkey neck and arm skin be damned.

## Buy Expensive Beauty Products (Or Don't) But Remember Where Your Worth Comes From

Listen, this isn't a knock on women who see the value in these products. I firmly (despite not being firm—see what I did there) believe that we all should do whatever makes us feel good. If you're a happier person wrapping your neck in skins that have been shed by rare snakes from Argentina, then girl, YOU. DO. YOU. And I'm not being cheeky. I really mean that with my whole heart.

But I do think that at some point, makeup and beauty products switch from something we do for fun and experiment with when we're young to something that hides what we really look like and tricks us into believing we're actually able to fight the aging process. And it's alarming that this shift is happening at younger and younger ages. Girls who are far from the glaring signs of getting older are already using filters in their pictures and are injecting anti-aging synthetic fillers into their faces. And, honestly, it breaks my heart when girls and women today don't embrace and value their "natural" beauty more often, especially young girls who really are the picture of youth. And especially older women who are truly radiantly gorgeous—gray hair, wrinkles, and all.

Personally, I have no interest in spending my money on products when I could, instead, spend my money on living life, seeing the world, and making memories that I hope will outlive me. But just like I want to do what makes me happy, so should you. (Full disclosure, I also never really learned how to use most of this stuff, so here I am, at 44, holding on to the remnants of whatever eyebrows are left after the Great Tweezer-gate of the 1990s, with absolutely no idea how to apply eyeshadow or what lipstick suits me best or how to pick out a "good" makeup brush. I'm a mascara and lip-gloss girl and that's usually it, which means it's probably a little easier for me to fight the good fight against beauty and anti-aging culture when I was never really in it anyway.)

With that said, I want to address the fact that the diet and beauty industry are 100 percent reliant on us hating what we see in the mirror. And that makes me sad. Sad, and angry, tbh. I find it so toxic and damaging to women (who WILL age because it's biologically impossible not to) and who come in all shapes and sizes (because it's biologically impossible not to) that billion-dollar industries rely—and THRIVE—on us questioning our own self-worth because we are getting older or have fat on our bodies. Especially because we need fat on our bodies to live, and getting older means we are alive. Both of these things are the ultimate goal: live a life worth living.

To me, having wrinkles and gray hair and sagging skin means that yes, I am in my mid-40s now. And I look like I am in my mid-40s. So, I am not going to spend money to look like I am not in my mid-40s. Also being in my mid-40s means I have a lot of years now to look back on with pride and see the life I've made. Being in my mid-40s means I have raised children into their teenage years and it means I have a marriage that has spanned decades (yes, plural). It means I have had years upon years of positive pregnancy tests and hospital births and family vacations and first days of school. It means I have watched all of my kids turn 12, two of them turn 14, and one of them start high school and start talking about college. It means I have experienced love, loss, pain, and forgiveness. I have experienced career paths take unexpected turns, seen friendships come and go, and bid farewell to people I love whose time on Earth has come to an end.

All of these life experiences mean I have lived a full life, and I have a lot more to live.

And when I'm 80, my skin will be far saggier than it is today—and probably on more than just my neck and arms. (I think my eyelids are coming next.)

But how beautiful will the movie reel be as I close my wrinkly eyes and look back at the journey? I hope I don't have a lot of regrets, but there's one thing I'm sure of: I won't regret having said "no" to the anti-aging industry when they wanted my money. I won't regret replying with a *"Thanks, but my turkey neck and I are doing just fine."*

## Notes on Chapter 9

*If you, like me, want to flip off the diet and beauty industry and unapologetically embrace aging as a natural part of life, here is something I do to practice it:*

I think about what beauty really means. Personally, I find myself captivated by strong women who exude confidence and joy. Whose lives are chock-full of adventure and perseverance and courage. Who belly-laugh loudly and whose energetic presence is felt throughout the entire room.

Sometimes, those women have makeup on, sometimes they don't. Sometimes, those women have worked hard to fight aging, sometimes they haven't. But sitting there, listening to them, soaking up their exuberance, the way they support other women, the way they share their wisdom and pull up the next generation of girls ... that's the beauty I aspire to have.

And it has nothing to do with how loose their skin is or how much they weigh or if their eyelids are a little on the droopier side.

Listen, I get it. We are pummeled—PUMMELED—by the diet and beauty industry our entire lives. They are very good at getting into our heads and convincing us that our worth is tied to looking younger and making our bodies smaller. They're quite good at it because that's how they make money.

I know how it feels when you see a beautiful, fit woman your age who clearly is all the things you're not. But here's what you need to remember: She's not winning the game of life because she looks 30 even though she's 45 anymore than you are. She might be the kindest, loveliest person on the planet or she might be a raging she-beast who is very alone and sad. Our wrinkles (or lack thereof) do not define us. If buying skin-firming cream makes you happy, buy it. Just like if getting a manicure makes you happy, DO IT.

But if you're hoping for a feeling of intrinsic self-worth after you've had Botox injected into your face, that's where things get tricky. Because you're likely looking into an empty well. Your beauty, worth, and value on this planet come from how you make others feel. How you treat your friends. How you raise your children to be kind, helpful, empathic, hard-working, and humble. How you sit with your grandma on Christmas and let her tell the same story she tells every year as if it was the first time she's told it and hold her hand.

That's beauty.

Because you know what? Someday that will be us. Someday we'll be sitting there on Christmas with our grandkids, hoping they'll listen to our stories, and we'll be the most beautiful thing in the room. And there's no magical serum the beauty industry can provide that can do that.

# Chapter 10

# On Friendships

If there's one brutal life lesson that hits you right in the gut at some point during adulthood, it's that true girlfriends are hard to come by. And that sometimes you have women in your life who you think are your "girls"—your ride-or-die besties. The ones who would not hesitate to pick you up if you fell. The ones who would, you have no doubt, be your loudest cheerleaders if you were to ever "make it big" in life. The ones who would *"fix your crown"* as true girlfriends promise to do.

And chances are, you're right. They'll be there—for the ugly parts and the beautiful parts and all the mundane parts in between. But also, they might not. And that's when learning life lessons sometimes, frankly, just hurts.

Because I've moved all over the country and haven't even stepped foot in the state where I grew up in well over a decade, I don't hang out with high school friends. In fact, I only even communicate with a couple occasionally on Facebook. And college isn't much better. I haven't made it back there in as many years, and with how busy everyone is raising babies (and now teenagers), it's just hard to keep in touch.

And, honestly, I've always been okay with not having the traditional "high school bestie friendship" or "college girlfriend reunion" so many others do. Because each place I've moved to over the years, I've made new friends—some ride-or-die girls who cheer me on in life and I know would undoubtedly "fix my crown." And some who were in my life for a time and simply aren't anymore. And most of the time that's okay and seems fitting for my busy grownup life as a mom of three.

But once in a while, the end of a friendship takes your legs out from under you, doesn't it? When you feel what you thought was a genuine connection with someone and realize after a few ghosted texts that, well, she's just not that into you?

## Breaking Up Is Hard to Do

I had a friend once who I thought was the real deal. She was in the same career field as me and newer to the scene. I felt immediately drawn to her due to her outgoing personality, incredible talent, and dry sense of humor I relate to so well. We crossed paths at conferences and participated in lots of group chats full of endless laughter and meme sharing as well as authentic love and support when one of us was hurting.

She was my friend. My close friend. Until I realized that she wasn't and actually hadn't been all along.

It was things like finding out she'd been randomly in my hometown and didn't try to meet up (and yes, she knew I lived there). Or going to a conference and finding out she'd roomed with someone else even though we'd always talked about bunking up together. But the big punch that took the wind out of me was when I had a big career moment—a dream publication that I'd worked hard for—and when I shared the news with her, there was no cheer, but rather a hint of bitterness. Jealousy maybe? Even though she'd also had her own share of accolades, for some reason, her heart didn't feel inclined to support mine. And, honestly, the most painful part for me was that she was one of the first people I told because she was someone who I always thought would, as girlfriend code dictates, *"be my biggest cheerleader."*

I've also felt the sting of a local mom friend doing the two-tier ghosting thing. You know what this looks like. You used to hang out a lot, and when you see each other, it's still great. Hugs! Smiles! Happy to see each other! But then one day, there aren't any more calls to meet up for drinks. And when you reach out, she's always busy and never reciprocates. You know you might still run into each other. And you know that likely nothing "bad" happened, but you also know it's time to let her go.

And, even as a grown-ass woman, I have found myself changing for others. Acting like something I'm not so I'd be liked, included, accepted, just like I did in middle school. Quieting myself when I think I'm being too loud. Agreeing with what other people say even though I vehemently disagree, but want to be "likable." It's jarring when you step outside of yourself and see what you've done. When you mentally float above your body for a quick second and see someone you don't recognize. You know you did dumb shit like that at 14, but at 44?! Come on. *"You're better than that,"* you tell yourself.

## Adulthood Can Actually Still Feel Like the Seventh Grade

> **21stcenturysahm**
> Teaching my kids to not chase down friends, & instead, give their time & energy to people who actively show that they want my children in their lives — this is one of the hardest parts of parenting.

I want to say that as a big old adult, none of this happens now. That stuff like this doesn't affect me anymore. That it doesn't hurt.

I want to say that I've grown all the way up and when I meet new people and feel a connection with a potential new friend, that I don't hesitate to reach out. I want to say that I jump right in, sending the message *"Let's be friends!"* because I'm not in seventh grade anymore and this isn't hard or scary.

I don't want to admit the truth: that I wait for what I hope is an appropriate amount of time before eeeeek! Hitting that "friend request" or "follow" button on social media. That I overanalyze those early connections, ensuring that I don't come on too strong and look creepy and desperate. And that I get nervous and excited and preemptively prepare for disappointment when it's someone I really like, hope she likes me, and think that maybe we can be friends and fill each other's cup. Especially if she's one of those unicorn friends who has a husband or partner my husband clicks with and kids around my kids' age that they can hang with, having similar interests. That's the real jackpot.

I want to say friendships are easy for me now. But they aren't. I hesitate, I overanalyze, and I stress about screwing it up and being left out of yet another group chat.

The truth is, I can't imagine my life without girlfriends. So, yes, it burns to lose one. It hurts to be ghosted. And the sting of having a "friend" turn out to be a competitor who resents your success can linger for a long time. However, I never stop trying to fill that painful void with someone new. Someone I can be my authentic self with and not go home and question everything I said. Someone who gets that I haven't always showered and I hate bras and I talk a lot. Someone who I can laugh with until my face hurts and cry with just as easily. That's it. That's pretty much my list. (A willingness to enjoy an adult beverage and snacks with cheese are a plus, but not a requirement.)

And when my kids go through the pain of losing a friend, being cut out of a clique, or being left off an invite list they thought they were definitely on, I want to tell them that it gets better. That the pain they are feeling is something that doesn't happen when they're older. But I'd be lying.

When one of my kids was recently mourning what seemed to be the end of a years-long friendship (not because anything bad had happened but simply because the friend had moved on and left my child in the past), I said, with honesty, that the pain will pass, and true friendships will help heal that wound. But I also had to say this is a part of life and an experience that each of them will probably experience again as teens and as adults.

And when another one of my children was chasing the glittery sparkle of the popular crowd and, as a result, seemed to be leaving some really good, strong, reliable friendships in the dust, we had to talk about that, too. Not only do we want to seek out real, authentic friends, but we also want to make sure that we, too, are real and authentic as well. That *we* are the tried and true friends others can turn to—to fix *their* crown. To cheer *them* on when they have a big moment. To help *them* stand back up when they've been knocked down.

In the end, all we can do is give our best to the relationships in our lives that mean the most and fill us up with love, support, and joy.

Thankfully for me, even in times of friendship deserts when I've just moved to a new place and I'm having a hard time cracking into tightly established friendship cliques, I still have a couple crown-fixing, ride-or-die besties who I know will always cheer me on and always pick me up when I fall. And they know I will never falter and will 100 percent do the same for them. These girlfriends may not live near me and I may not see them often, but they are there.

And they'd never show up in my hometown without knocking on my door for a glass of wine.

---

## Notes on Chapter 10

***The takeaway on this one is short and blunt:***

You have to let go. Grieve, feel the hurt, let yourself sit in it for a bit, but then let them go. We cannot expend energy chasing fake friendships, and we cannot watch idly by as our kids expend energy chasing fake friendships either.

If someone isn't authentically showing up for you, you have to let them go.

If you are not your true self when you're with them, you have to let them go.

If you don't come away from spending time together feeling full, and instead feel depleted, you have to let them go.

If they aren't genuinely happy for you when something good happens in your life, you have to let them go.

No one is going to say it doesn't suck, but it's the only path. You deserve better. Your kids deserve better.

That's it.

# Chapter 11

# The Comparison Trap

The comparison trap doesn't discriminate. Like guilt, this toxic game seeps into our lives at an early age. We learn to compare ourselves to others as kids—and, unfortunately, to measure our self-worth through those often false comparisons.

When we were young, there was always that girl in school: the one with seemingly effortless beautiful hair, naturally smooth skin, whatever "body type" was most coveted during that decade, and a confident, outgoing personality. It's nearly impossible for impressionable children to not compare themselves to whatever "ideal" society has created for the time period. What really hurts the psyche, though, is deciding that we are "less than" in some way because we're not her.

Eventually we grow up and grow out of such dumb, pointless comparisons. (Hahaha, no we don't.) Women—grown ass women like myself—still do it. There's still "that girl" only now she's "that mom" and she's at school picking up her tiny mini-me—a younger, perfect version of the girl we all knew years ago.

This mom has it all together. The fit body, the money for expensive trends in clothes, shoes, and jewelry. Her hair is done. Her nails are done. Her makeup is done. Everyone wants to be her or at least be in her inner circle.

You, on the other hand (and by "you" I mean "me") haven't showered today (and maybe also not yesterday either). Your hair is not done. Your nails are not done. Makeup? Where even is your makeup these days? You're wearing an old baggy sweatshirt you found in the back of the closet and yoga pants you've had for a decade (you've never done yoga). And when your kid opens the door in car line, a McDonald's soda cup falls out onto the curb. Perfect mom definitely doesn't feed her kid McDonald's.

She glances your way, offers a weak smile, and your face burns in shame. Somehow, you've let this other mom define your value. (FYI, she has struggles—we all do—even if our challenges are hidden.) You let the comparison trap win, again, just like when you were a kid.

And it's not just what that perfect mom looks like. It's the vacations she takes and the car she drives. It's her should-be-on-HGTV immaculate home and her perfect marriage to a gregarious partner named Bill, "who LOVES to cook!" What a great guy that Bill is.

You hate her. And you hate how much you also want to be her.

Because even though you're giving every drop of everything you have to your family, your kids, your spouse, your home, your job, and whatever and whoever else needs anything from you, you've now reduced yourself to dust because of the comparison trap.

It gets all of us, so don't beat yourself up if this story sounds familiar. But do know that there are ways to combat this toxic mindset.

## Comparing Ourselves to "Perfect" Moms

I've learned about the damage the comparison trap can do firsthand because I'm not immune to it—not at all. And more than the yucky feeling moms get when comparing themselves to another mom's looks, my toughest battle is measuring myself against how other mothers, well, mother.

The single greatest struggle of motherhood, for me, has been fearing that I'm not doing a good enough job. So, when I would see a "gentle parenting" mother speak calmly to her kids at the playground, I'd feel like a failure, knowing full well that I already lost my shit that morning because the kids couldn't find their shoes *"which should be in their shoe cubbies but heaven forbid anyone ever put anything away around here!"*

Or the summer bucket list moms. They got to me every summer for years until I finally learned to let it go and reevaluate how I looked at *my* summers with *my* kids. So we didn't make a bucket list and go on daily nature walks to collect pine cones for a craft. Some days, we just watched a lot of screens or just played outside in the yard with the hose because Mom didn't have anything else to give.

**The 21st Century SAHM**
@21stcenturysahm

Kudos to the summer bucket list / daily adventure moms—you're amazing.
But to all the moms who find those lists to be too much pressure and whose kids are sleeping in, watching Netflix, reading books, and riding bikes up and down the street all summer, you're amazing too.

But every summer, I'd look back and realize I could make a list, too. Throughout June, July, and August, we went to the library, we hit the park, we swam, we played outside, we rode bikes, and we ate popsicles. Just because we also watched a boat load of *Paw Patrol* and sometimes ate fruit snacks for breakfast doesn't mean I was a bad mom. My kids had fun and made memories, just like the kids who had bucket lists did—we just forgot to write it all down.

Or how about the back-to-school moms who are legit sad and say they're going to miss their kids? Or the *"You only have 18 summers! Cherish every minute!"* moms? Do you compare yourself to them? I do.

Because honestly, the *"Thank God summer is over, please get on the damn bus, goodbye love you lots"* mom? That sounds more like me. Because the truth is, I do treasure the summer memories we make. But I'm sure not sad when school starts either.

And whether you mourn the end of summer or you skip with joy as your kids head back to school, you're a good mother too.

Listen, there are a million ways to be a good mom. Not every SAHM is going to be a bucket-list mom who "goes on an adventure!" every day of the summer months and cries when school starts. For one, leaving the house is expensive, and staying home is not. Also, some mothers are pregnant or just had a baby or are fighting chronic illnesses or disabilities or their kids have special needs or they are in the throes of a mental health battle and their depression and anxiety is crippling.

And some moms (and kids) are perfectly happy to live a simpler life of crafts at home, free play with dolls, and collecting as many colors of rocks as they can from the creek behind their house. Sometimes that's all the "adventure" they need.

Measuring your success or failure as a mom against another mom's social media feed or the way she "gentle parents" when her child talks back in public or pees their pants in the cart at the grocery store is a surefire way to drive your self-worth right into the toilet. Look at your kids. Do they love you? Do they feel your love? Do they feel safe? Do they smile and laugh? Do they get excited to show you the flower they just picked or bring you invisible tea and cookies from their play kitchen? Then your list is complete. Check it off: *"Good mom."*

> **The 21st Century SAHM**
> @21stcenturysahm
>
> The other day I spent a couple hours with a good friend who was fighting back tears because all her kids are now in school & she misses them so much it hurts.
>
> I danced down the driveway with joy as my kids hopped on the bus.
>
> We are both good moms.

## The Working Moms vs. SAHMs Fight—STOP DOING THIS

Unfortunately, another common area for comparison is the SAHM vs. working mom battle—a battle I HATE with all of my soul because every single mother I know, whether she goes off to work every day in heels or stays home in sweats, loves her children fiercely and works tirelessly from the moment she opens her eyes until the moment she finally allows herself to rest at night. This festering comparison infuriates me and is so damaging to mothers everywhere because no one wins in the end.

But yes, when we're prone to comparison anyway, it isn't a huge leap to the next level where you compare your unshowered, haven't-used-a-brain-cell-in-months self to the professional mom in a power suit across the street. Or flip the script: That mom may see you pushing your kids on the swings and feel pangs of guilt that she was gone all day, missing all the opportunities you had to spend time with your kids. Both might feel like the other is "better" or "worse" when really there's no comparison at all. We're all good moms.

When the comparison game seeps into your bones (it's probably already there), you have to look at the big picture of your life as a mom and your kids' lives as children. You have to find the small moments of joy, the trips to the library, the surprise cookies in the backyard, the snuggles at bedtime, the time your toddler twirled and squealed with joy in her new princess dress, the time your five-year-old learned to ride a bike and yelled with pride, "I'm doing it, Mommy!"

And then you take a breath and say, "I'm doing a good job."

## Notes on Chapter 11

*I have learned a thing or two over the years about how to stave off the toxicity of the comparison trap, mostly because I've been stuck in the muck enough, and I had to climb my way out. Here are my tips (there's a lot here so buckle up):*

1. **Practice gratitude.**

    First of all, gratitude is one of the most powerful tools to fight negative thoughts. Gratitude has helped my marriage (see Chapter 18), it has helped me fight resentment when I'm carrying the mental load (see Chapter 7) and yes, it helps reframe my thinking when I find myself comparing.

    It's really very simple, and it's all about mindset. For example, if I come home to my messy house with old, stained carpet and jelly smeared on the counter, and I had just been visiting with a friend whose house is clean and freshly renovated where none of the counters are sticky, I remind myself of a few things. First, oftentimes, friends of mine who have houses like that have children who are grown, and they have told me time and time again how much they miss it. How quiet their house is now. How they'd give anything to go back and have a day of kids crashing on the couch, eating snacks, laughing, and leaving their shoes everywhere.

Also, I have friends who have faced infertility battles and don't have kids or maybe have one and desperately wished they could have given them a sibling. When I feel overwhelmed with my home and feel angry at the messes in every room, I am reminded that there are five of us—five people I am grateful for every day.

And finally, remember this: although you're envious of what someone else has or looks like, someone else is envious of you. Someone else out there would give anything to have your marriage, your home, your beautiful children, your life.

2. **Make a list (I talk more about this in Chapter 3).**

   When you feel down about yourself and feel compelled to compare your "mothering" skills or any other aspect of your life to someone else, you have to choose what you're going to focus on. Which list matters more?

   If you're comparing yourself to some "perfect mom" who does it all, has a clean house, exercises, spends time with her kids, nourishes her marriage, has a thriving career, volunteers at school, and is entirely happy and fulfilled every minute... Well, first of all, acknowledge the fact that she's not real. That person doesn't exist.

   But, also, remember that you likely do all (or most) of those things too, just not all at once. So, reread Chapter 3 and make the list. The first one. Then flop into bed at night knowing that you were successful today in lots of ways. And tomorrow's another day.

3. **If you're going to compare, reconsider who you are comparing yourself to.**

   I was talking to my therapist recently about how my current fitness regime and my husband's don't match. He's on a big health kick and whipped himself into shape (with a ton of hard work) and I'm still, well, me. I work out, eat healthy-ish, and still look like a regular mom who works out and eats healthy-ish.

She noticed right away that I was comparing myself to him, which will not serve my mental health in any way. His journey is his journey, and I can support him and cheer him on, but I'm on my own journey, too. She reminded me that I have been "working on myself" for years. I have been in therapy, addressing my anxiety, and practicing body positivity and acceptance for myself and for my daughter to see as an example.

When I have an hour of free time and I choose to sit in the quiet and read a book, that's me taking care of me.

When I try to drink as much water as I can every day (even if it means I have to pee every 42 seconds), that's me taking care of me.

When my workout is walking the dog and listening to a podcast I'm excited about, that's me taking care of me.

When I go out with my girlfriends and drink wine and eat fried cheese and laugh hysterically, that's me taking care of me.

Those are the pieces of my journey. And whatever my body looks like right now, I need to feel proud of all of the ways I'm taking care of it.

Also, if you're comparing yourself to *yourself*, be wary of the tendency to think about "how skinny you once were" or "how young you once looked." I've been guilty of this, too, and here's what I try to remember: 25-year-old me was skinny and young and FUN. But 44-year-old me is stronger and wiser than she was. 44-year-old me has pushed out and raised three phenomenal humans. 44-year-old me has traveled the world, made two new decades of memories, eaten delicious foods, drank delicious drinks, and laughed until my face hurt. And she's worked through pain and forgiveness and learning a shit-ton about herself.

So, yes, I'm bigger than 25-year-old me. And I'm older. You can see it. But I'm also wiser, braver, and stronger. And I think 25-year-old me would be damn proud of who I turned out to be.

# Chapter 12

# The Water Challenge (and How We Need to Reframe "Success")

I talk a lot about failure (see Chapter 15) and how my crippling fear of it has caused me to unintentionally put up roadblocks throughout my life. But what I've learned about words like "*failure*" and "*success*" is that they really are defined by how we frame them within the context of our story.

And an epiphany about something as simple as a personal challenge to drink more water helped me realize this.

I've been in a Facebook workout group for years—I think maybe going on a full decade. I don't live near any of these women anymore, having moved away long ago, but we've kept the group going as simply a source of accountability. We check in after we've done some self-care ("*Lifted weights!*" or "*Took dog for a walk on this beautiful day!*") and we have many times in the past embarked upon challenges like a plank challenge to get to our own PR, a pushup challenge to do 100 pushups a day for a month, and even a water challenge to drink 100 oz per day.

I've done the plank challenge many times (personal record is three minutes!); I've done the pushup challenge, doing them in batches of 10–15 because that's my body's pushup max (why are pushups so damn hard?); and I've attempted the water challenge pretty much every day for the past few years, but that one has proved, surprisingly, to be the hardest to achieve. Maybe it's because I birthed three gigantic babies in five years and live in the "need to pee" state 90 percent of the time, so drinking 100 oz of water in one day means I'm on the toilet more than I'm not.

Maybe it's because, a couple years ago, we got a pandemic puppy and now I'm basically a toddler mom all over again. Therefore, if my hyper, needy dog is finally sleeping, I will do everything possible to not wake him up, including getting up to pee (or get more water).

Maybe it's because every weekday from 4–9 p.m. and during the summer months and on spring break and winter break and teacher work days and all the other random days the kids don't have school, I morph into an Uber driver and live in my minivan. (Again, making that whole "need to pee" thing a challenge.)

Maybe it's because after the kids leave for school, I finally sit down at my computer with my first sip of coffee and then spend the next few hours praying the dog naps, throw in a load of laundry, meal-plan, check the family calendar, run the dishwasher, sit back down to write some more, and at some point realize I still haven't had breakfast (or a drink of water) and now it's nearly noon.

Whatever the reason, I almost never succeed at getting all the way to 100 oz. I've gotten close but all the way to 100 oz in a day? Nope.

I guess, every time I don't make it to my goal, I fail ... right?

Or how about this?

Every time I say to myself, "I'm going to drink 100 oz of water today," *I win.*

Every time I try to do something good for my body, *I win.*

Every time I don't quite make it but I can look back knowing I did my best for myself and that I'm going to try again tomorrow, *I win*.

Every time my kids see me taking care of myself and I physically feel stronger and healthier, *I win*.

I mean, isn't this how we talk to our kids? Don't we tell them how there is beauty and glory in the journey? How, if they don't make the team or don't get into their dream college or even if they fail a math test, there is still success in trying their best? If our children work hard at their sport, craft, or future career goals, there might be times along the way that things don't work out—but that doesn't mean they've utterly failed and should give up. That just means they should reevaluate their system, tweak their plan, or pivot to take another path, but that they need to see all the success they've had too. Hard work is success in itself.

We have to do better at talking to ourselves the way we talk to our kids.

This is an important mindset as we think about what we're going to do when the kids grow up. When we aren't driving them 9,000 places between the hours of 4 and 9 p.m. or all day long in the summer. When we finally have time to prioritize other things that are good for us (not just water).

If we set goals for ourselves and work really hard to achieve them but fall short, we can choose to look at ourselves as failures for not getting there. Or we can see ourselves as winners for trying and getting back after it the next day. Maybe we realize that whatever goal we've set needs adjustment. Perhaps this isn't the right post-mom-life career path. Or you might feel a calling to do something else. Maybe this journey doesn't fulfill you in the way you'd hoped. Or it could be that it's just really hard to achieve and you're exhausted and need rest. Or maybe you've resolved to keep going after it, chipping away at that proverbial giant cup of water every day.

In any and all of those scenarios, you're winning, not losing. You might feel like a hamster on a wheel, taking tiny sips and wondering if you're going anywhere, but you have to step off of the wheel and look at the bigger picture. You're doing something for you. You're taking on a challenge, whether it's a self-care challenge or a career challenge or a personal challenge to write a book (talking to myself there). Keep taking those sips and keep going.

(No matter what, though, drink more water today! It's good for you. Am I a self-care life coach now?)

## Notes on Chapter 12

***How to reframe success in your life:***
Think of your life and your goals like a giant cup of water. Last week, maybe you only drank 30 oz of water. Today, maybe you drank 50. Tomorrow? You might hit 60! Sure, you've yet to reach 100 oz, but look at you—you're doing it.

What does your "100 oz of water" look like? A physical challenge like training for a race? A professional challenge like going back to school or embarking on a new career path? A mental or physical challenge like starting therapy or new medication or a commitment to eat healthy?

Whatever it is, if you're doing it, if you're trying every day, despite setbacks, and you chip away at that goal, getting closer and closer, you're showing your kids what a winner looks like. Nobody ever succeeded by taking the easy path. The only way to really get a place of true "I did it! I did the really hard thing!" is to take the more challenging road. It's about standing back up each time you stumble and getting back on the journey after you've taken a step off for some much-needed rest or time to heal.

If you're doing that, you're already a success.

# Chapter 13

# Get Thee to a Therapist!

English teachers and readers of Shakespeare know the famous line from *Hamlet*: "Get thee to a nunnery." Well, I'm sure nunneries are lovely (I wouldn't know), but I'd never tell a woman to go there unless she wanted to. I *will* tell you—all of you—to get yourself to a therapist STAT. And I *will* continue to advocate for women and mothers seeking out help, seeking out someone to talk to, seeking out someone who can help them break through the walls they've built up throughout their lives and who can help them figure out why the walls are there in the first place.

Everyone talks about self-care and making sure Mom gets a break and can take a long bath or sleep in on the occasional Saturday. All good stuff, all good stuff. I'm a big fan of moms getting rest. But here's what else I'm a big fan of: learning about who you really are. The greatest gift you can give yourself is dissecting all those inner parts of you and then putting the pieces together to complete the picture—a picture you can step back from and be like, "*Ah, yes. Now it all makes sense. Now I understand why I lost my ever-loving shit last Tuesday when I found a dirty cleat on the counter.*"

One of the reasons I write is because motherhood has been 1,000× times harder than I ever imagined it would be. Having children and being a mother was a yearning I'd felt my entire life. Some girls, like my teenage daughter, aren't sure yet. Maybe they'll have kids, maybe they won't. But I knew. I knew at four years old when I'd lovingly dote on my baby dolls. I knew as a teen when I'd snuggle the little ones I was babysitting, dreaming of the day I had my own.

I got engaged at 23 ... *"When can we have kids?!"*

Married at 25 ... *"When can we have kids?!"*

And finally, the day I'd dreamt of my entire life, at 27, I saw a positive pregnancy test for the first time. It was going to be magical and everything I ever wanted. I believed that with my whole soul.

And that's why it was crushing for me when I didn't love every second of it. That's why I felt like such a dismal failure when being a SAHM to babies and toddlers wasn't fulfilling, and in fact, made me resent my husband even though I had the life I'd always dreamt of.

It wasn't until I cracked open the shell of me, with the help of a therapist, that I figured out who I really was. It wasn't until then that I began to learn why motherhood was so brutally hard on my mental health. And how I could work towards a better, stronger me—for myself and for my family.

I know that accessing effective, meaningful therapy isn't feasible for everyone for lots of reasons, so I thought I'd share some things I've learned about myself. Things that have helped to explain many of my struggles, especially in the early baby days, but even now, as a mom of teens and tweens. And, maybe, by sharing my stories, I might be able to help another mom out there with similar struggles.

## Five Truths I've Had to Accept About Myself

### 1. I need to feel smart and intellectually stimulated

I was a high school English teacher who loved my career, and I worked until the day before my first child was born. That meant the adjustment to motherhood was abrupt, not only because I was suddenly in charge of keeping a tiny human alive who had just emerged from my body into the world but also because I quickly went from being in a large, busy, noisy building surrounded by students and colleagues and meetings and lesson planning to a quiet little apartment with just me and a newborn who struggled to eat.

And, immediately, I felt myself falling into a dark place, but I didn't know why. Surely if I was only busier (read: had more babies), I'd find that magical *"loving every minute 100 percent fulfilled"* idyllic picture that had lived in my head all those years while I dreamt of being a mom. So I did. I added two more babies. And still, the darkness persisted.

It wasn't until I actually started writing and establishing a new career—my own career—that the sun began to shine again, and now I know why. I do understand that my job as a mom was the most important thing in the world. It still is. But changing diapers and washing sippy cups and folding tiny pairs of pants didn't make me feel smart. And the more days that passed without intellectual stimulation and challenge, the more resentful I grew.

Talk therapy has helped unearth this truth about myself, and my only regret is that I can't go back and find new-mom-me in those early baby and toddler days, get a computer in her hands, and start sooner.

### 2. *My perfectionist brain makes me feel like a failure a lot*

Motherhood and perfectionism are like oil and water—they'll never mix harmoniously (see Chapter 15 for more on this). I didn't know that going in (nor did I know how much my need for perfectionism controls my brain) so I fell flat on my face from the get-go.

Over the years, I've worked hard to let a lot go, like my house being clean for example. But it's a choice I have to make every day. When someone in our house makes a mess (literally, or figuratively by making a bad choice), the perfectionist in me starts to panic.

"Oh no," it says. "Everything in our world isn't neat and tidy!" and I have to talk her down. I have to remind her that no one else has the perfect life either. And that I'm still a good mom because good moms work through the messy bits and come out on the other side stronger and wiser.

And this makes me a better parent because not only will I make mistakes, but guess who else will? My kids. I have teens and a tween right now and this age is ripe for the picking when it comes to errors in judgment, selfishness, and not thinking things through. That means life gets messy sometimes, even when you've got good kids like I do.

### 3. *I need alone time and personal space like I need oxygen*

Having had this need met throughout my life before becoming a SAHM, I didn't know how crucial it was to my well-being. Although I'd never lived alone and had hopped from an apartment with my college girlfriends to an apartment with my future husband, I still had regular periods of quiet, of alone time, and of personal space. But that all stopped when I brought a few new humans into the world who would gnaw on me, climb on me, and invade my bubble every minute of every day for over a decade.

It's why I sometimes feel like crawling out of my skin.

It's why one more noise sends me to my breaking point.

It's why I joke about hiding in the closet with a snack (but really, I'm drowning and want to cry, not laugh).

It's why, on that last day of school in June, when my kids hop off the bus and rejoice that "*It's summerrrrrr!*" in cheery Olaf voices, my stomach churns as I try to feel joyful for them. And it's why I feel like a crappy mom when I don't cherish every day of those three long months because, as we're incessantly told, "*We only get 18 summers with our kids!*" (Even though that's a lie because I'm 44 and spend a good chunk of summers with my parents.)

But, yes, having now endured 16 years of being home with my kids, I know how this story goes. The anxiety of sensory overload and lack of quiet alone time begins to crawl up my back, wrapping itself around my shoulders. I painstakingly orchestrate moments of quiet alone time and undoubtedly, a child will come careening around the corner and interrupt my moment of peace. And especially when it's that same child who also left their dirty clothes on the bathroom floor and breakfast dishes on the kitchen table, well, that's when the volcano erupts.

This is just a truth about me I have to accept. And while this need for quiet alone time is met regularly during the school year, the months of June, July, and August create a recipe for anger and negativity. A recipe I must counter (and now that I have older kids, this is easier to do) by leaving the house, going to a coffee shop, and finding a chair in the corner where I can work, read, or zone out and not hear one of my kids gripe about our lack of chips or whine about having to walk the dog.

We can only do the best we can do with the strengths and shortfalls we're given. But I hope that when my kids look back at their childhood, they'll say, "*I had a good mom. She was a writer. She didn't love summer as much as other moms, but she did her best. She was there for everything. And we always knew how much she loved us.*"

## 4. I have anxiety (and sometimes anxiety makes a person look like an asshole)

In an unexpected turn of events, recognizing my son's mental health struggles helped me see my own. My third child's anxiety has manifested itself into anger. When he doesn't have control over a situation (like when his shirt was itchy as a toddler or, as an 11-year-old, when his hockey stick almost broke because his older brother put a heavy backpack on top of it), he goes from a calm baseline to an anger level of 100 in seconds.

And while it's not acceptable to flip out and let our anger control us, it does help to understand the underlying cause.

As I learned more about him and his emotional triggers, I started to see myself. When the house is a mess and I don't have control, I flip my shit. When I can't get everything done that I want to achieve and I feel overwhelmed, I lose it. I become angry and mean and the entire household feels my negativity.

Knowing this about myself (and about my child) has helped me address the anxiety first—which, in turn, means I can address (and help prevent) the anger that happens as a result. (I talk more about this in Chapter 15, too.)

**5. *It's okay to not love it all—I'm still a good mom***

This one is big for me. I have to give myself permission (still, after 16 years) to not love it all. Because, holy shit, there are moments in motherhood that no one loves. No one loves blowout diapers in Target. No one loves when toddlers pee on the floor at church. No one loves functioning on 2.5 hours of sleep. And no one loves arriving at a long-awaited park playdate that both you and your toddler so desperately need because he needs sunshine and exercise and you need grownup conversation (even if that conversation is interrupted 92 times) only to realize that he's not wearing shoes and you're 30 minutes from home. (Yes, that happened and yes, I cried.)

> Listen Carol, I know I'm supposed to "enjoy every minute" while my kids are young, but right now one is crying because another one called him a toilet face, so why don't you come hang out for a few hours and let me know if YOU enjoy every minute.
>
> – The 21st Century SAHM –

No one loves these moments. But we're told we should because "*it all goes by so fast.*" And they're right—it does. My high schooler was that toddler at the park without shoes like five months ago (it seems). I'm well aware of how fast it goes, but moms in the trenches also need to hear that it's okay to not love every moment.

In fact, it's okay to downright detest some moments.

That doesn't mean you're failing. Or that you're not a good mom. Good moms look around, say, "*Well, this moment royally sucks*" and maybe even have a little cry in the car. But they wipe their faces and keep going because they know there are beautiful moments ahead.

I mean it. Get thee to a therapist if you can. (Mine also hates summers! Hearing her say that was so damn validating.) Learn about yourself. Learn to give yourself grace and forgive yourself. Or if therapy isn't in the budget or there's no option on the mom-calendar, be your own therapist. Figure out what you need. Don't wait until you're six years and three kids into parenting to start figuring things out. Be your own cheerleader. Write yourself notes and stick them to your mirror.

"*You are strong.*"

"*You can do this.*"

"*You are a good mom.*"

Because all of those are true and you might just need a reminder.

---

## Notes on Chapter 13

### *How to learn about yourself:*

Obviously, a professional therapist will help here, but there are other ways to learn about your core needs. Because if a darkness has settled over your days as a mom, chances are, one or more of your needs aren't being met.

They might sound dumb, but taking a quiz to find out your "love language" or what "enneagram number" you are might truly help you learn about, well, you. For example, learning how highly I prioritize praise (super high—like top billing) was instrumental in realizing why the early motherhood years were such a challenge.

I had gone from a career where I had regular assessments and frequent "good job!" type message from my superiors to a continuous rotation of diaper-changing, breast-feeding, and potty-training with zero accolades. And I needed them more than I realized.

Having learned that about myself earlier in my motherhood journey could have saved me (and my husband and my kids) a lot of stress as we fumbled through the muck, wondering why Mom was having such a hard time.

Also, talk to the people in your life who know you and whom you trust. Ask them what they know to be true about you, and be ready to hear their honest answers. Are you competitive? Do you accept constructive criticism? Are you a perfectionist? Are you an introvert or extrovert? Do you have anxiety that controls a lot of your thoughts and behaviors?

Learning about WHO you are will help you understand WHY you are the way you are. And from there, the floodgates will open and it will all start to make sense as you work towards a happier, healthier you.

Finally, even if you struggle (we all do), you're still a good mom. Write that on a Post-it and stick it to your mirror.

# Chapter 14

# Of Course We're Pissed Off

Nothing pisses me off more than being asked why I'm pissed off. Really? Let me change out of this sweaty shirt and I'll tell ya. Pull up a chair and get comfy because there's a list.

First of all, we've been fed a toxic lie since we were in preschool (see Chapter 3)—a lie boys aren't told. Boys and men are pushed to work hard, have careers, support their families, and get used to ticker-tape parades every time they do the bare minimum that girls are expected to do. Push a stroller? Gold medal! Change a diaper? Dad of the Year trophy! No one asks them how on earth they cope with the guilt of leaving their kids to go to work. No one tells them they're shitty dads if their kids are outside without a coat or drink formula as babies. They can't possibly worry about such things! They're too busy and tired from working hard at their careers all day.

Women and girls, on the other hand, are told we, too, can have careers and dreams and that *"We can do all the things boys can do!"* Even better, we can also push out babies! Lucky us.

Yes, lucky us, truly, because it is a blessing. Bringing my three children into this world were the proudest moments of my life. But what no one told us when we were growing up, dreaming of *"what we wanted to be"* alongside the boys was that even as the babies came, their careers and dreams and aspirations would continue to sail up, up, up into the sky. And ours? Some of us would never leave the ground again. Some would skip across the sea for a bit, treading water here and there, and a few would take off and shoot for the stars, but they'd dodge meteors for the rest of their lives as mothers. Meteors men somehow already have armor for.

No one told us that mom guilt would feel like 900-pound weights on our shoulders, holding us down from sailing alongside our male counterparts at work. No one told us that we'd have to rush back to work well before we were healed, before we were ready, before our babies were ready, because our employer wasn't obligated to hold our position for us, or pay us while we recovered, and we actually should be grateful we got any maternity leave at all in this country.

We're pissed off because society has set us up.

As young girls, we were fed a glittery picture full of dreams, but once we got to the gates, ours opened up to endless more doors we'd have to knock down and locks we'd have to decode while our brothers and husbands and fathers and sons were able to walk right through.

We're pissed off because their path stays smooth and shiny, while ours derails into low-level jobs that allow us to carry the mental and physical load of motherhood. Mothers who want successful careers see hurdle after hurdle and are instead often pushed into toxic multi-level marketing businesses that prey upon women and only drive wedges between mothers who should actually be supporting one another.

We're pissed off because we know we deserve more, we want more, but we can't figure out how to manifest the extra hours we need to achieve greatness at a job we've been working toward, a job we've invested our education in, and a job we're actually good at while also being the kind of mom we want to be and the kind of mom the world expects us to be.

We're pissed off because society tells us we're shitty moms if we don't give up any and all career goals and instead, revel in the joys of potty-training and washing out curdled milk from the inner parts of unnecessarily complicated sippy cups. No one expects dads to find joy in these tasks.

We're pissed off because despite doing 7,612 jobs daily, we're asked what we do all day.

We're pissed off because we're judged regardless of what kind of mom we are.

We're pissed off because today's mom is expected to get on the floor and play with her kids...

*While also taking care of herself and hitting the gym ...*

*While also nurturing her marriage and friendships and family life ...*

*While also feeding her children natural organic foods ...*

*While also maintaining a clean home ...*

*While also monitoring her children's screen time and exposure to the evils of the internet ...*

*While also staying up late to be available for when her teen unexpectedly wants to talk ...*

*While also volunteering at school and making sure assignment notebooks get checked and reading logs get signed ...*

*While also adding money to the E-Wallet so her kid can buy books at the book fair ...*

*While also remembering to take the dog to the vet ...*

*While also scheduling time to get her oil changed because that annoying light has been on for two weeks ...*

*While also making sure she's not a helicopter parent but still somehow knowing where her kids are every single second because if something happens everyone will click their tongues and way, "Where was that child's mother? Was she ignoring him and staring at her phone?" even though there's a 874 percent chance that she's on her phone scheduling an* orthodontist appointment for that child or researching dinner ideas because the pediatrician mom-guilted her about calcium and fiber and also because everything she's made for the past 10 years other than frozen chicken nuggets is met with whining and zero gratitude.

And she has to do all this while smiling! and "*not getting emotional*" even though hot-headed men have been having temper tantrums, throwing insults, and starting wars since the beginning of mankind.

So, yes, we're pissed off.

Also, we're pissed off because our bodies have endured monumental physical and hormonal shifts for the past three to four decades without rest. And in that time, we've also grown and pushed out some new humans into the world, who then used our bodies as chew toys in the middle of the night, and pawed at us throughout all the daylight hours as well. And, for extra funsies, despite being the literal reason the human race continues on, we're also fighting for our rights (and our daughters' rights) to even make our own decisions and choices about our war-torn bodies that have been out there, on the front lines, doing all the things, for 40-something years.

We're hot and sweaty, our backs hurt from carrying our families literally and figuratively every day of every week of every month, year after year, and we're exhausted because when we lay our heads down at night, our minds continues to race, replaying everything we need to get done tomorrow that we didn't get done today and everything we need to remember to get done the day after that.

And despite all that, we're told that our worth is diminished because of a wrinkle or a few pounds or a spot of cellulite on our thighs.

We're pissed off because, yeah, we gave it all up—the career, the control over our own bodies, the freedom to spontaneously grab lunch again for a full decade, the personal space—partly because we wanted to and partly because society measures mothers based on how much they're willing to sacrifice.

And now we're ready to have a turn, our turn. We did it all and we don't regret it for a second, but we're wondering now what's next for us.

But we're not sure if there's a place at the table for 40-something moms who've lived in sweats for 15 years. When we try to claw our way in, we're told we're *"unqualified"* or *"don't have enough experience."* We have our *"resume gaps"* questioned even though we've been doing 1,000 jobs at once on zero sleep for years on end.

So, please, stop asking us why we're pissed off. Just move over and let us through. We've got shit to do.

---

## Notes on Chapter 14

***If you're pissed off, good. That's a start.***
Now channel that anger to vote for women's reproductive rights.

Vote for better paid maternity leave.

Vote for better maternal health care.

Support women in leadership roles who are out there, on the front lines, who know first-hand what it feels like to be pissed off about all the things on this list, and who are working for change.

Join local organizations—big changes happen locally. Get involved with your local school board or town council.

Volunteer for your county or state representatives who believe in making the world safe, fair, and equitable for women and girls.

Let's stay pissed off until the job gets done.

# Chapter 15

# Anxiety, Perfectionism, + a Crippling Fear of Failure = a Toxic Cocktail that Does Not Mix with Motherhood

I started getting chronic migraines at eight years old. They run in my family (my dad was plagued with horrendous headaches as well) so maybe I had no chance at living a migraine-free life due to simply my DNA.

But eight years old is quite young to be hit with the barreling train of frequent mind-splitting pain, loss of eyesight, and vomiting—genetics be damned. My mom did ask the pediatrician what also could be causing these regular migraines that ravaged her little girl's tiny prepubescent body?

"She's stressed out," he said.

Stress. At eight. Third grade. What were the great "stresses" of 1988? Hmm let's see: Was it wondering if I would get the Barbie

Dream House for Christmas that year? Or if my bestie Lauren and I would score 50 cents from our parents so we could get Creamsicles from the ice cream man? Or how I'd spend my afternoon—riding bikes or climbing trees? How would I decide?

It was absurd. How could this skinny little New Kids on the Block–loving third grader, with a safe and stable home life, be "stressed out"?

But now, at 44, I can look back and see all the puzzle pieces come together. Third grade was the first time I had to navigate real friendship drama as there was a girl in my class who didn't like me and made it her mission to ensure no one else liked me either. Third grade was the year my bestie since birth (who lived across the street) moved far away, to another state, leaving a giant hole in my childhood heart. And third grade was also the year I got my first "B" on a report card. It was the first time I could remember being less than perfect. It was the first time I realized I didn't have control over everything. And it turned my whole world upside down.

That year—my eighth around the sun—was just the beginning of a lifelong fight against anxiety, perfectionism, and a crippling fear of failure. A toxic trifecta that 20 years later, I'd only truly realize was dominating my entire being. Because two decades later was when the biggest thing to ever happen in my life took place.

Newsflash (this is not a newsflash at all): If there's one thing that does not mix with anxiety, perfectionism, and a fear of failure, it's motherhood.

## When Motherhood Enters the Chat

I had my first child at 28, which meant I had 20 good, strong years in there fighting the good fight. Coping with migraines, overthinking every single interaction with friends, and as I got older, overthinking every interaction with boyfriends, coworkers, college roommates, new adult friends; 20 years of living in relentless fear of messing up, of not excelling in school, of saying the wrong thing; 20 years of analyzing my ever-changing body, obsessively working out and counting calories as a teen, cleaning my tiny 600-square-foot apartment as a young adult, making sure everything was perfect. Making sure I was perfect. (Spoiler: I never was.)

Before motherhood, I anxiously tried to achieve perfection in my career as a teacher, poring over lesson plans for hours upon hours at my tiny kitchen table.

Even on my wedding day, there was only one option, and it was as damn-near perfect as any wedding could be, down to the off-white (not white-white!) cocktail napkins. The makeup, the dress, the flowers, the church. Perfect, perfect, perfect, perfect. So perfect, in fact, that I struggled to actually enjoy the day as I was too busy obsessing over what I now know are insignificant details.

I had spent my life as a perfectionist always trying to attain the unattainable but never wavering in my mission because failure, of course, was not an option. And when you're a perfectionist, anything "not perfect" is a big fat fail. There's no middle ground.

And after living this way for the past couple decades, I obviously only had one track in mind for this next phase of life. I mean, I was going to be the perfect mother with the perfect baby obviously. Why would anything else be acceptable?

However, we all know how this really goes and that, in actuality, motherhood would just push me further along on my anxiety-laden, driven-to-perfectionism-to-the-point-of-exhaustion track.

Nothing knocks a would-be perfectionist off her horse like pushing out a baby. It happens swiftly and it happens painfully. And suddenly the solid footing you've always relied on is lava and you're feeling things you've never allowed yourself to feel before ... I think they call it ... (whispers) "failure"?

It took three hours of pushing and the use of a vacuum that gave my baby a cone-head to get my first-born out. FAIL #1.

He wouldn't breastfeed. FAIL #2.

I didn't love every second of motherhood from the moment the nurses laid his tiny wrinkly body on my chest. FAIL #3.

And they just kept coming. Fail, fail, fail.

Potty-training at two years old? Nope. We were peeing our pants well past three.

Immediate bond with his new sister who arrived two years later? Not a chance. He asked us politely to "please send her back."

Endless patience and days filled with stimulating, educational activities that completely fulfilled me because motherhood was something I'd always wanted? Ummm more like a depressed mom who wondered what in the hell she was thinking because this shit was 1,000× harder than she'd ever imagined and she'd obviously made a huge mistake (three times, actually) because she sucked at this. All of it.

Fail, fail, fail.

## The Noise of Anxiety

The anxiety reared its ugly head on a near-daily basis because I had no control. I couldn't make my kid pee in the potty any more than I could make him eat a carrot. He was a whole human with the capacity for his own thoughts and opinions. And he was two years old, so a lot of those thoughts and opinions were irrational.

And it grew into an even uglier anxiety-monster because I wasn't perfect. I was, in fact, so far from perfect that I didn't even recognize myself. My formerly spotless house was always sticky and smelled like curdled milk. My fit 20-something self had been stretched and torn and bruised and battered and simply wasn't mine anymore. But the worst part was having to accept these lapses in perfectionism. I didn't know how to be less than perfect and how to see myself as anything other than a terrible failing mother.

Also, anxiety, for me, is noisy. And because I didn't realize until well into adulthood (see Chapter 13 and learn about yourself!) that I was fighting this constant battle, I'd simply just learned to live with the noise in my mind. Wasn't everyone's brain like this? My husband says that it often seems like there are bees buzzing in my head and holy cannoli is that accurate.

It was already pretty damn noisy in there with lots of stressed-out buzzing, and then motherhood entered the chat.

Because motherhood truly is that one powerful force that will take all your preconceived notions about how you think life is going to go and it will toss all of those pieces into the fire.

Oh, of course, you'll get pregnant (it won't be hard to do that!) and then you'll enjoy nine months of blissful excitement (nothing will go wrong!) followed by the breeze of breastfeeding (my body will know what to do!) and the serenity of holding my sleepy baby (he'll sleep, right? RIGHT?!) and eventually the joys of first steps and tiny feet toddling across the kitchen (not breaking anything of course! Not MY child!) and you'll love it all.

Every. Single. Minute.

You won't be bored or unfulfilled or desperately miss your career or miss having a reason to shower and wear cute boots again. None of that will matter! It will be okay that your boobs hurt and your belly looks like the dough your grandma used to make bread out of because THIS IS WHAT YOU ALWAYS WANTED, SO YOU'RE ONLY ALLOWED TO BE GRATEFUL.

Even if you feel anxious. Even if you feel yourself folding inward, shrinking, disappearing because, if you can't be the mom you thought you'd be, you wonder if you should even be a mom at all.

## But Wait ... What if None of That Is True?

What if you're not a failure and you're actually a freaking fantastic mom whose kid just happens to not want to breastfeed or potty-train until 3½?

What if good moms can be anxious moms, and anxious moms can be good moms all at the same time?

What if you're a work in progress, you're slowly letting a lot of your rules go about how clean the house is, and that maybe it's okay if you and your baby wear clothes with spit up on them to church?

Then maybe, just maybe, someday you'll be a 44-year old mom of teens and tweens and you'll know 100% without a doubt that nothing and nobody is perfect and that you are a really, really good mom to three kids who God made just as they were supposed to be.

And, equally important, you'll realize that whatever this next chapter of your life brings after your hashtag momlife days are behind you, that you can and will find success despite the failures you'll encounter along the way. You'll understand that whatever it is—a new career, a business venture, a big risk (or even a small risk), a new set of goals, dreams, and aspirations (all of which you 100 percent deserve), you'll know and accept that it won't be perfect. But it will be pretty freaking great because you will be doing it.

## Notes on Chapter 15

**If you're a recovering perfectionist with anxiety and a crippling fear of failure, welcome! Let's be friends. Repeat after me:** *"None of us is perfect and we all fail. You're a good mother."* (Write that on a Post-it and stick it to your mirror.)

Now, take the power away from anxiety and perfectionism by naming it.

*"This is the anxiety talking."*
*"This is the perfectionism talking."*

Naming it takes away some of its power and paves the way for other thoughts. Once you've named the anxiety and perfectionism, then say to yourself, "I don't have complete control over everything. It's okay if this isn't perfect. I'll get through this."

And finally, do these things to quiet the buzzing:

- Take five deep breaths.
- Do something that soothes you like listen to music, meditate, go for a walk.

- Make a list of everything you need to get done. Come up with a plan. Talk to your partner and kids about what you need so everything gets accomplished.
- Control what you can and talk yourself through accepting all the imperfections of what you cannot.
- Will you succeed every time? No, sometimes the buzzing might win for a bit. But sometimes it doesn't. Sometimes, you'll win and you'll quiet your mind. Then you can remind yourself that you're doing a good job, even if every corner of your life isn't neat and tidy and wrapped with a bow.

Also, here's a relatable tweet for my anxious friends:

> **The 21st Century SAHM**
> @21stcenturysahm
>
> That panic attack you have when you suddenly realize you're not panicking about anything so clearly you must have forgotten to do something because there's zero chance you have all your shit together

# Chapter 16

# Learning to Get Out of My Own Way

In 2019, I ran a Ragnar Race with my husband, a few of his sisters, and some friends. If you know me in real life, you know that I am zero percent athletic. If you know my husband and his sisters, you might know that their family is uber-athletic and competitive in a friendly (*read: not always friendly*) way. And if you're familiar with the Ragnar, you know that it's for people who really enjoy self-punishment like running in dark woods at 2 a.m. and not being able to walk, sit down, or get back up for a week. Each person on our team (including me, the non-runner, non-athlete) ran three different races: a 4-ish mile loop, a 6-ish mile loop, and an 8-ish mile loop. Some of those were run midday. Some started in the middle of the night.

When my husband and his sisters first brought up this idea to me, inviting me to join their team, I immediately WITHOUT HESITATION said absolutely not. I cannot do that. I'd run a few 5K races over the years (slowly) and one 10K that damn-near killed me. But this beast? Not a chance in hell.

And that's when my husband said something that I'll never forget. He asked me why. When I said, "*I can't,*" he responded, "*Why not?*"

"*Because ... because ... because I just can't,*" I stammered, having no other explanation.

"*Says who? Who says you can't?*"

Well, fuck. It was me. I was the only one saying I couldn't do this race. And it sucked to realize how much I doubted myself. So, I made the decision that day to get out of my own way, train my butt off, and join their team. We wrote out a training plan, starting with just running a mile or two. And it was hard. By the end, my longest run before the race was an 8-miler through our town. It took FOREVER and I think a few people literally walked past me because I'm slower than a turtle crawling through molasses. But I walked (limped) in the door that night and said to my family with pride, "*I just ran 8 miles!*"

I was still scared though. Running the Ragnar meant taking one- to two-hour naps in a tent, getting up, strapping a headlamp to my head, and setting off into dark woods in the middle of the night. Ummmm. WHAT? And yeah, I had done that single 8-mile run, but then I sat on the couch, icing my knees, calves, and pretty much everything else and watched *House Hunters*. At the Ragnar, I'd have to run, rest, run again, rest, and then run AGAIN. I still didn't know if I could do it.

Eventually, the day came and we drove out to the middle of nowhere Wisconsin to set up our tent. It was go-time.

In the end, did I run it? Yep. The whole freaking thing. Was I the slowest person on our team? Sure was. And did everything hurt so badly that I nearly cried for days after? Like you wouldn't believe.

But I'll tell you what—I've never been so proud of a physical accomplishment. I've told myself my entire life that I can't. "*You can't ___ because you're not athletic. You're not a runner. You're not this, you're too that.*"

Nobody else has ever told me that I can't. It was me all along. And when I stopped saying it, when I got out of my own damn way, I overcame an incredible physical feat I never believed I could achieve. I ran the Ragnar and have the medal to prove it.

And now, here I am again, getting out of my own way.

## Becoming a Writer ... Again

I've wanted to be a writer since I was six years old. By eight, I was writing novels in my bedroom. Everywhere I went as a kid, I asked for paper and a pencil so I could write a story. My parents still have the hand-written tale *"Mystery on Cave Island"* that I think is like 10 to 15 chapters long. I wrote it as a child, bound it with yarn, and slapped hand-drawn cardboard pieces on the front and back. It was my first "book"—one of many, I thought to myself back then.

At some point along the way, however, that dream turned to dust and floated away on a cloud. I changed life paths and embarked upon a teaching career—one that I loved dearly. I was a high school English teacher, which meant writing was still a substantial part of my life. But the writer in me? She seemed to be long gone.

Until she resurfaced about 25 years later.

One day in early 2011, not long after my second child was born, I told a story on Facebook about how going to the grocery store with a boogery toddler and a newborn pooping through her clothes was an adventure. A few friends loved the post and said, *"You should be a writer!"*

I think something woke up that day from a long slumber. I shouldn't BE a writer. I AM a writer, I realized. I always have been. I was just on a two-decade long detour, that's all.

So, I started, and over the past decade and a half, my writing career has flourished. I've been published on endless parenting sites as well as in several anthologies, and my social media following has grown. And as I delved deeper and deeper into my dream career as a writer, the idea of writing a book always loomed in the back of my mind. But as is my standard MO, I kept holding back.

"*You can't write a book,*" the voice in my head told me (no one else said it). And the years ticked by.

Until the writer in me resurfaced yet again—the *book* writer this time though. And, ironically, it all started from yet another social media share just as it did 14 years ago.

This book was born out of a Facebook post I wrote in the fall of 2023 that resonated with mothers everywhere—a post about realizing we didn't know what we were all going to be when our kids were grown. As I watched the responses to that post grow and grow, I started thinking, "*This is it. This is the book.*" But even then, that toxic self-doubt held me back, and I didn't take the leap for a while.

A few months after I wrote that post, one of my closest friends said to me, "*You should write a book. Every time I read something you write, I feel like you're talking to me.*" And although lots of friends and family members have told me that same thing over the years, for some reason, her comment stuck. Maybe that's because I was finally ready to get out of my own way.

I felt a nudge that day and took one step out. "*Maybe I can actually do this,*" the voice in my head started to whisper. And I started talking to some writer friends about how they got started.

A short time later, I heard a song on the radio that gave me my final push. That Facebook post about wondering what we'll all do when the kids grow up reminds me of the Martina McBride song "This One's for the Girls," specifically the line "*This is for all you girls about 42 ....*" Every time I heard that song after I had written that post and saw how successful it was, I'd belt it out, feeling pride in how I was reaching so many women and mothers out there, like me, who were in their 40s, watching their youth slip away, wondering what comes next. And one day I turned the corner to drive up my street and sure enough, there was Martina, helping me along with the shove I needed.

I remember laughing and saying, "*Okay, God. I hear ya.*" And that was the day that "*You can't do it*" voice shut the hell up, and I finally sat down and started writing all of these words.

It was all of these pushes—some big, some small—writing that Facebook post, feeling encouraged by a friend, hearing Martina McBride on the radio: Each one has nudged me along. These small moments have taught me to stop doubting myself, to stop standing in my own way. And, finally, I guess I just realized how much I wanted it—even if it meant it was going to be hard and I might stumble at times.

Despite, getting good grades, graduating with honors, and even having the success in writing that I have had over the years, I have struggled to believe in myself my entire life. It's much easier to say, "*I can't*" because then I don't have to possibly face failure. My fear of not being perfect (see Chapter 15 if you haven't yet—it's a doozy) has kept me snug and secure in my safety net where I don't have to take risks.

*What if I write a book and no one reads it?*
*What if I write a book and people DO read it?*
*What if I'm not perfect and some people don't like it?* (I talk about this more in Chapter 28.)

All of those thoughts were enough to keep me solidly, directly, in my own way until I finally mustered up the courage to believe in myself.

It may have taken a decade and a half since I wrote that first blog post about going to the grocery store with my tiny humans to actually write a book, but I did it. I eventually got the hell out of my own way.

So, here it is.

And when I stepped off the path and finally let myself through, do you know who I saw when I turned around and looked back? There she was—childhood me, standing there, pencil in hand.

And here's my promise to her: As I figure out what I'm going to be when the kids grow up, I'll make sure to keep the path clear this time.

---

## Notes on Chapter 16

**It's time.**

The takeaway here is pretty clear. Get THE HELL out of your own way. Especially now, as you're nearing the next chapter of life when you aren't as tethered to mothering tiny people. Now, when your kids are now taking all of the life-lessons you've instilled in them and they're flying off, doing life, being their own grownup selves.

If there was ever a time to look back and revisit old dreams, it's now.

If there was ever a time to dust off any regrets and "I wish I had …" thoughts, it's now.

But you have to step off the path and stop being your own roadblock.

You have to be willing to fall, to fail even.

You have to be willing to write a book that people might read (or not). A book people might like (or not).

You have to be willing to run a race through the woods in the middle of the night with a head lamp. (Okay, maybe not that exactly, but you get what I mean.)

It's scary. I know. I'm several panic attacks in already as I get ready to hit publish on this sucker. But I'm doing it.

Are you doing it?

# Chapter 17

# Nobody Talks About the Loneliness

I've said it repeatedly throughout this book, and I'll say it to anyone who will listen. The greatest gift we can give ourselves (and, subsequently, to our relationships with others) is to learn about who we are. What our core needs are. What we thrive on, and what breaks us down.

And, honestly, I think that the abrupt adjustment to parenthood (which really feels like being launched into a lava pit) is so hard for relationships because the adult(s) in the room don't know a lot about themselves. We think we do: "*I'm good at sports*" and "*I like to read!*" but when someone hands us a slippery baby to take home that we're supposed to raise into a kind, contributing member of society (a responsibility that feels like 5,000 pounds), the truth comes out of who we *really* are.

I thought I knew the kind of mom I was going to be. I had been dreaming of having kids my entire life which obviously meant I was going to be super good at it! I was going to have endless patience and feel entirely fulfilled and find immeasurable joy in every moment! Of course that's how it was going to go—I'd wanted this for so, so long.

And when it didn't, when I didn't feel super good at it, when I ran out of patience, when I didn't feel fulfilled and downright disliked parts of motherhood, everything turned bleak fast.

Honestly, I wish we could better prepare new mothers for how crushingly lonely and boring it can be. How you communicate all day to a tiny blob who doesn't respond and how you're kind of like Tom Hanks talking to a ball on a deserted island.

And then you put the baby down for a nap and you think, I should call my mom, my girlfriend, or my sister, but you don't because you'll have to pretend that everything is fine and that you're fine.

*"Yes, the baby is doing great"* you'll have to say, but really you want to cry out, *"I miss the world and happy hour and freedom and buttoning my pants!"*

But that would make you ungrateful and unappreciative of this blessing, so you soldier on in silence and then your husband calls to say he'll be late tonight and the resentment grows as the needle on the clock just got moved farther out.

For me, a few vivid memories stand out—ironically, because they were about simple errands or just going outside for fresh air with my baby or feeding him in a quiet room at a family event. Just regular days, at the grocery store, sitting in my yard, or nursing my hungry baby for what felt like the hundred thousandth time. Why do these seemingly mundane moments in time represent so much of early motherhood to me? Because this was my life. The simple, the repetitive, and the feeling that I was, more than anything, alone.

At the time of these memories, I was a mom of one tiny baby—the child who, in many ways, got the best of me and the worst of me as a new mom. Our days were long, quiet, and lonely. Maybe not for him, but certainly for me. And I still haven't quite forgiven myself for not loving motherhood more when it was just two of us.

I'd worked as a high school English teacher, analyzing *Julius Caesar*, *The Poisonwood Bible*, and *The Canterbury Tales*, until the day before he was born. I was grossly unprepared for the drastic shift between spending my days in a big building, bustling with noise, having endless tasks to complete and constant conversations with students and colleagues alike, to hours upon hours at home in our little apartment, with one sleepy newborn and me.

We'd go out, desperate to break up the day. But going "out" was no small feat for a new mom who was struggling to breastfeed and feared a blowout diaper in public. That meant one "outing" a day was really quite enough for this struggling mother.

## The First Holiday Season

The first memory of realizing just how cripplingly lonely I was happened at a family holiday party. I became a mom in November, which meant visiting with extended family and introducing my newborn to everyone on both Thanksgiving and Christmas that year. Both holidays were joyous and exciting, providing opportunities to show off my adorable son in some cute and super impractical outfits like khakis with collared shirts and tiny brown boots.

But the memory of that holiday season also has a cloud of isolation and loneliness hovering over it, as I spent a large chunk of the family gatherings in another room, breastfeeding my cluster-feeding child. Again, just my baby and me all alone.

I can remember listening to the laughter and merriment on the other side of the door and desperately longing to be a part of it all. Desperate to be back in the world where grownups were and people spoke to me and asked me questions and challenged my brain.

The truth is, of all the adults at a holiday party, there's probably no one who needs to be in the room more than a lonely mom of a new baby. But sadly, she's the one missing.

Because our first child struggled to breastfeed, but was finally getting the hang of it around this time, I had committed 100 percent to nursing (and to not risk the possibility of nipple confusion with a bottle). And because he never fully relaxed and got a full feeding in each time, that meant he spent the first few months of his life feeding every couple hours.

There I was, a new mom still learning how to properly feed with a baby who was still learning how to properly feed. A new mom who couldn't fathom doing it in public yet. There were too many factors: I needed my boppy, a roomy chair, and the ability to focus and work together with him without distraction.

But all that meant that my husband and entire extended family enjoyed Thanksgiving and Christmas in a way that I did not. And in a way that I desperately needed.

## An Invisible Friend Down the Street

One of the most telling examples, to me, of just how hard those early newborn days were was that I had a girlfriend five houses down the street who had a baby two days before I did. She was FIVE HOUSES AWAY.

Guess how often we saw each other? Almost never.

Despite my painful loneliness I didn't call her, and she didn't call me. I think we were both afraid of saying the truth out loud. We were probably both so scared that the other one was doing great, loving every minute like she was supposed to. Not missing our careers and wondering why the hell motherhood was so unlike what we'd dreamt of our whole lives. Instead of commiserating and getting together and telling the truth, we stayed in our own houses, alone with our shame. (At least that was my story and why I didn't call her.)

But honestly, what if she was doing great and loving it and her baby was feeding well and she didn't stare at the clock all day? I couldn't bear the thought of it, so I stewed in my own loneliness instead, for fear of her (and the world) finding out the truth.

## A Bright, Sunny Day

Another vivid memory that still brings a pang of regret and shame to my heart was on St. Patrick's Day of 2009, when that same baby was a few months old. We were living in Wisconsin, so March is a gamble on any given day, but the sun was out, and it was warm enough to spend some time outside.

"Well, that's what we'll do!" I thought, optimistically. "We'll go outside and enjoy the sunshine and, well, we will figure it out when we get out there!"

I brought a big blanket and some baby toys, and out we went, to sit in the front yard and the fresh air.

And that was it.

"Okay ... what now?" I asked myself (and my four-month old child—he didn't offer many suggestions).

"Should we go for a walk? Well, he needs to eat soon, so probably not," I told myself.

Instead, we sat there, looking at each other, looking out at the street, and then we went back inside.

It was 10:15 in the morning, and I didn't know what else to do with my day.

"*This isn't how I thought it would be,*" I thought to myself.

## Where Were the Other Moms?

Fast-forward a few months. We were no longer living in that tiny apartment but now a real house—our first house—with lots of room to play and grow. But the rest of the story is pretty much the same. We'd moved to Kansas, and I knew no one. But it was okay! We purposely moved into a cul-de-sac and became suburbanites (which I had never thought we'd do), and my street was obviously going to be chock-full of other SAHMs, right?! I couldn't wait to meet them and have friends. My long, lonely days were about to change, and I was ready.

Once we were unpacked and my husband was off at his new job, ready to take on the world, I, too, was eager for this next chapter. On another beautiful, sunny day, I popped my little baby into his stroller and off we went, ready to find all the other mothers in the neighborhood who were as desperate as I was for some grown-up interaction.

I walked up and down the street and saw no one. It was quiet, just like the inside of my house. And eventually, we just went back home. It was St. Patrick's Day all over again.

So far, motherhood had been nothing like the idyllic picture I'd dreamt my whole life. I didn't feel super good at it, nor did I feel immeasurable joy and complete fulfillment every moment. All I knew was that even though I was doing the most important work of my life and had an absolute blessing in my arms, I felt so very alone.

I spent my days looking at the clock and counting the number of hours until another adult (my husband) was going to come in and save me from this emptiness, at least until the next day. And I hated myself. I resented my husband for being in a big building with endless conversations and important tasks to be done, and I felt unbearable shame when I looked at my child—a child I'd dreamed about having since I was five—that I didn't love every moment with him.

I just never thought motherhood would be this lonely.

## Standing in the Bread Aisle at the Grocery Store

Yet another memory of those early baby days was a trip to the grocery store. I'd timed it, so as to best break up the day—don't go too early in the morning but don't wait too long into the afternoon. "*This is good, something to do,*" I pitifully told myself.

And it was good, for a while. We talked as I walked the aisles, me telling him what colors were on the cans: "*green*" for green beans and "*red*" for pasta sauce. Passersby waved at him and told me how cute he was.

Until the second to last aisle, when it hit me that we were almost done.

"*Surely we're not almost done,*" I said to myself. "*Maybe I forgot something. Maybe we should walk through all the aisles again.*"

And the shame and embarrassment I felt in that moment nearly brought me to my knees. I didn't want to be done yet. I didn't want to go to the checkout because that meant we had to go home, to the quiet, to the loneliness, back to staring at the clock, to the realization that I was really, truly struggling and not the mother I thought I would be.

I can remember that day very clearly because it was so emblematic of my first two years of motherhood. Adding another child (and then another) didn't necessarily make all of the demons go away, but the house wasn't as lonely, and it definitely wasn't quiet anymore. Mostly, the loneliness was just replaced with chaos and sensory overload, but that's another chapter entirely.

But that mom who hated how much she struggled with this job that she'd wanted her whole life? Even after the third baby, she was still there.

The woman with a master's degree, who graduated cum laude, who, just a few months ago was grading character analysis essays and setting up debates in her class on climate change was now standing there, staring at rows upon rows of bread, praying that when she got home, it would be 2:00, not 1:00, so that she had one less hour to fill.

*"What have I become?"* I thought to myself, feeling every part of me shrink into the void. Everything I knew about myself had dissipated, and what was left felt like a failure. I had the cutest, sweetest little child right there with me. A little boy with a tiny voice who loved books and trains and puzzles and who could never give enough hugs. I was his whole world from morning until night, and I didn't see it. I couldn't see the sunlight through the clouds over my head.

I was doing my best, but simply getting through the day. That was the best I could do, for him.

## If I Could Go Back

Now that my tiny newborn who struggled to breastfeed is a teenager taking Drivers Ed, I look back and feel a lot of sadness and regret that the clouds above were so dark and hung around as much as they did.

I see social media videos of moms holding their tiny babies, reveling in their giggles. I can see sheer joy in the mothers' faces and oh, how I sometimes wish I could go back. I wish I could find new-mom-me so I could tell her a few things. I'd hold her face in my hands and make sure she heard me as I said, "*You're doing a good job. It gets better.*"

And maybe if I could relieve her of some of that anxiety and guilt and shame about "*not loving every minute*" and feeling lonely when she held the greatest gift on the planet in her arms ... maybe if she just heard that she was doing okay then she could look up and feel a bit of sunshine on her face. Maybe she'd have been able to find a bit more joy as the hours ticked by.

But I can't. All I can do is look at the amazing humans I have raised and know that even when the world went dark as it so often did, I kept going. I did my best. We figured it out together. And eventually, the sun came out.

## Notes on Chapter 17

*It really is lonely sometimes.*

This chapter was hard to write. Looking back at those lonely early baby days unearthed a lot of old pain, and I'm still working on forgiving myself for how dark it all was. But I wanted to tell this story because I know without a doubt that mothers out there are feeling this same loneliness. Even though everyone has smart phones now and social media, there's a mom out there, looking at the clock, wondering how in the hell it's only 10:15 in the morning, and hating herself for thinking that thought.

I want to tell her something she needs to hear—something I needed to hear. It's really boring sometimes. It's lonely. You're still a good mom. You're doing a good job. It won't always be this way.

Also, this is an important chapter for moms who are past the baby days but are heading into the next phase and are wondering what they'll do, who they'll be. I want us to remember how hard we worked, how much we sacrificed, and how strong we are for having gotten through it all. And then I want us to say, "It's my turn now" and go out there and grab a hold of something that is ours for this next season in our lives.

Finally, if you're a lonely mom wondering how you'll get through the day (in whatever phase of motherhood you're in) and you have a friend down the street, call her. She's probably hoping you do.

# Chapter 18

# How Resentment and the "Who Has It Harder" Game Nearly Killed My Marriage, and the Daily Phone Call That Probably Saved It

I heard once that as much as support and understanding are pillars that hold up the foundation of a marriage, resentment is the thing that will kill it. It is toxic, damaging, and does long-lasting harm. It seeps into the cracks of your relationship, worming its way through any slight instability in those support beams, and threatens to burn everything you've built to the ground.

And it's true. Resentment (on my part) damn near killed our marriage.

*I resented my husband swooping in to be "fun Daddy" after a long, tiring day of mothering for me.*

*I resented that because he hadn't been with them all day, he always had more of himself to give the kids while I was perpetually running on the last drop in my cup.*

*I resented when parenting seemed easy for him and he'd say "The kids were great!" on the off chance I'd escape for a few hours.*

*I resented that my work always seemed invisible, while his job was deemed "important."*

*I resented when people would say that he "worked so hard" but not say that about me.*

*I resented when he'd tell me about a fancy work dinner where he was served lobster mac & cheese while I ate cold chicken nuggets my kids had left on their plates.*

*I resented him leaving for work in a suit or an ironed shirt while I spent the day in his old sweatshirt from college that was now covered in baby spit-up.*

I used to get dressed in expensive pants and ironed tops for work. I used to eat fancy dinners and drink cocktails at happy hour after work on Fridays. And yes, I had chosen the path of a stay-at-home mom, but I couldn't fight the feelings of resentment.

I knew I was lucky—yes, even blessed. I knew that many mothers wished they could stay home with their children but they couldn't afford to not earn a paycheck. I knew how fortunate I was, but I missed my old life. I missed feeling important and smart and professional. I missed grownup conversations and challenging discussions. I wanted to switch places some days and have him stay home, wiping jelly off the floor and practicing letters with an ABC puzzle. I wanted the chance to call and say I was eating a fancy dinner and having a glass of wine at a rooftop bar or that I was going to be late because I was still working on a project.

And for all of those reasons, resentment had seeped in. And it was killing us.

The hard truth is that for all its blessings, parenthood really puts a marriage through the ringer. Having a tiny needy baby pushes parents to the very brink of their mental and physical capacity, and because you're both tired beyond measure and have not a single drop left to offer, you find yourselves playing the "Who Has It Harder?" game—a game with no winners and a game that is a toxic cocktail for a relationship.

But oh boy have we played it.

Who has it harder? The parent who has to get up at 6 a.m. every morning, get dressed in professional work attire, and face the pressures of bosses and clients and colleagues barking at you all day while you face the immense responsibility of knowing it's on you to feed your entire family and pay the mortgage?

Or the parent who was up three times breastfeeding the previous night and will spend the entire next day feeling sticky hands pawing at her while she continues to nurse all day long, tries to get the toddler to pee IN (not near) the potty, attempts to get the laundry done as everyone is out of clean underwear and socks, does the meal planning and grocery shopping (praying the toddler doesn't poop himself in the freezer section like last time), and also spend quality time with the kids doing things "good moms" do like nature crafts and "sensory bins" (which really just sound like a nightmare to clean up).

The first parent doesn't get a break all day long.

The second parent doesn't get a break all day long.

They are both exhausted and doing their very best, but because life depletes their tanks on a daily basis, they often have nothing left to give one another at the end of the day. And when one tries to vent about how hard their day was, the other might, rather than offer empathy, instead counter with, "Oh you think YOU had a hard day?"

And round and round they go.

The truth is, there's no competition. There's certainly no winner. There's just the daily grind of parenting little ones (which eventually becomes the daily grind of parenting teens, but that's another chapter for another day).

But for me, being so deeply engulfed in SAHM depression, loneliness, and guilt for not loving every minute and not feeling complete and utter fulfillment with playing pretend "store" and wiping tiny butts and wiping up the floor after bath time day after day, I was entirely blinded by how hard things may have been back then for my husband.

When you're drowning, it's hard to look over and see the person who might be right there with you also searching for a life raft.

And that's why resentment is so damaging and why it shoots often irreparable holes into the supports that hold up a marriage. Resentment clouded my view and led me down an even darker road—a road where I struggled to feel joy for my husband's accomplishments and empathy when he faced something difficult.

The truth was, I was jealous. I wanted to fly around the country on airplanes and have a beer over midday lunches and have an excuse to shop anywhere other than the sale rack at Target.

But it was more than that. I was jealous because I knew that he felt smart everyday. He felt needed—and not in a *"I'm keeping tiny humans alive"* kind of way. Although yes, I was doing the most important job of my life. I missed being needed as a professional.

Looking back, I realize now that neither my husband nor anyone else threw me a life raft (I needed to figure that part out on my own). But, yes, although we eventually hit the bottom of the ocean, we thankfully looked up, saw a beam of sunlight, and kicked our way to the surface.

And, honestly, I think it's the little things that saved us—seemingly small gestures that patched those fractures my resentment caused. One of those gestures was a daily phone call my husband has made to me almost every day for the past 16 years. And here's the backstory of why I think he made that call …

## What's for Dinner?

We had nearly a full decade of doing life together before bringing a child into our family, so he knew some truths about me that weren't going to change, SAHM or not.

One of those core beliefs (that I had stated many times over our early dating and married years) was that being a 1950s housewife was not happening for me. We were a partnership and both carried all the burdens of grownup life together. Early on, I had full intentions of being a working mom. He knew how much I loved my career as an English teacher, and we'd worked independently but side-by-side toward our respective futures throughout those years. During our post-college 20s, we both worked full-time during the day and attended grad school at night. In later years, he was a full-time student while I supported us as an educator.

And throughout those formative years of adulthood, while we were figuring out how to do life on our own, he did most of the cooking. For one, he was great at it—a natural in the kitchen. Also, he hated doing dishes and I didn't mind. We'd meal plan together, walk over to our local grocery store a block away from our cute second-floor apartment, come home, and grill up steaks or try new recipes like Cajun shrimp tacos.

But when I entered the SAHM-realm, it was a strange, but sensible transition to have me be the primary on meal planning and cooking. By this point, he was working very long hours. And I was home all day, looking for activities to fill our days, grocery shopping included.

But here's what he got right because he knew me so well. Every evening, as he left the office, he called home. But never once did he ask what was for dinner.

Instead, this is what he said and still says to this day, a decade and a half later: *"Do we have a dinner plan or do you need me to pick something up?"*

It was a small, but meaningful act. And it showed me that he understood that even though I was a stay-at-home mom, making sure dinner was ready every night wasn't solely my responsibility. Even though I was generally home most of the day, my days were as full as his were, and, more importantly, my work was as valuable as his work.

Never once, despite how absolutely destroyed our home was when he walked in the door, did he question how I spent my day. Never once did he question why something didn't get done, like the laundry, or the cooking, or the grocery shopping. If the kids were clean and happily playing, great. If they were greasy and covered with mud and there were socks hanging from the ceiling fan, he kissed me hello and scooped them up for hugs and snuggles.

And I know it sounds idyllic, but that doesn't mean it was an easy life.

SAHM life for me, especially during those early baby and toddler years was a grueling grind of guilt and self-hatred as I realized that I did not, in fact, love a lot of moments. It was the exhausting push and pull of feeling desperately alone but also completely touched out as there were tiny people in my personal space every second of the day. It was nothing like I'd dreamed and I channeled all of that negative energy into resentment toward the one person who was my partner in everything.

It took a lot (as in many, many) years to figure it all out. Why was I angry and jealous? Why did he not know what was going on with me? Why didn't *I* know what was going on with me?

I guess bitter resentment and overwhelming mom guilt about feeling like you royally suck at SAHM-life leaves no room for self-reflection in your mind.

## A Lifeline

The epiphany came after our second child was born and I started writing and seeing my work published. When I started saying sentences like, "*Mommy has work to do*"—oh the power of that sentence and taking my computer to another room to write an article. It was like I had put myself into a rocket and flew to the moon. Even though I was only writing a few articles per month those first few years and making almost no money, it felt like everything.

I felt smart again. I felt needed on a professional level. Sure, there were still no fancy dinners or justification for Ann Taylor clothes (that still hasn't happened), but it was something beyond wiping sticky fingers and cutting off peanut butter sandwich crusts. It was something to hold onto—a semblance of the former me.

It was like I had reached back into the portal and pulled her through even just for a few moments a week, and the reunification of old me and new me, was exactly the healing I needed.

And that's when the clouds of resentment began to clear. When my husband and I began kicking our way to the surface, eventually ending up on shore, breathless and tired but united in commitment to our kids and to one another.

Motherhood, for all its blessings and joys, can also be a dark hole pulling at one half of you while the other half frantically fights to break free. For me, the only way to make sure I didn't become fully consumed by such a powerful and dark gravitational force was to find something that was just mine. Something outside SAHM-life. Something that made me feel smart and important.

It was writing that saved me. And I know now that it was also a million other small things that probably went unnoticed but are noticed now.

And I'm pretty sure one of those small things was my husband calling every day to ask, *"Do we have a dinner plan or do you need me to pick something up?"*

---

## Notes on Chapter 18

*If you're in the trenches and you and your partner are spitting fire at each other or are more distant than ever, let me tell you a few things:*

1. This is normal and common. The baby and toddler days are brutal and you're unprepared. We all are. Give yourself some grace. There is nothing wrong with either of you. You're surviving learning how to be parents.

2. It gets better. I promise. Someday, they'll sleep all night (which means you'll sleep all night). Someday, your boobs will return to normal. Someday, you'll have the mental and physical energy to get dressed up and go out and have fun again—together. Like a real date. With romance. Really, you will.

3. If you're plagued with resentment like I was, learn from my mistakes and try to figure out which of YOUR needs aren't being met. Then figure out a plan to fix it so you can clear out the negativity and make room for the support, love, and kindness that you need to give each other to get through this. Are you someone who needs alone time in order to function? Do you miss being a professional? Do you miss your girlfriends? Are you just simply exhausted and need a weekend away to sleep? (See Chapter 13 for more on learning about yourself.)

4. Write this down on a Post-it and stick it to your mirror: "We'll get through this."

# Chapter 19

# Lessons for My Kids (and for Myself) as We All Grow Up

A huge chunk of parenting includes growing up right alongside your kids. Especially that first child and if you have more than one, they're the one who teaches you how to be a mom, just as they are figuring out how to be a kid in this world. I tell my first-born all the time that he's our first pancake. We're going to mess up a bunch with him—probably overcook him and undercook him all at the same time—but eventually we'll figure it all out together. Lucky him, I guess!

And now, as he and his siblings are getting ready for the next chapter in their lives, I've realized that we're still growing up together—just in a new way. While our teens and tweens are figuring out their next steps (how to be an adult, how to start off on their own, how to handle big responsibilities like driving, having a job, or even just learning to stay home alone), we, as moms, are figuring out our next steps, too. We have to figure out who we'll be when the SAHM chapter closes. And what we'll do with ourselves when there are no more calls from the school nurse, no more orthodontist appointments, and no more "*Mom, can you pick me up?*" texts.

We're growing up—all of us. Moms and kids. And here are some life lessons I hope my children take with them as they march into their teenage and young adult years. But as I have done throughout all the other chapters in this book, I'm also talking to me and reminding myself to keep these valuable pieces of advice close to heart.

## Six Life Lessons for My Kids (and Me)

### 1. Seek and foster real, authentic relationships in your life

Don't chase people down. If they don't show up for you, if they don't want you in their life, or don't care if you're there are not, leave them be. Spend your energy on friends who actively fill your cup, not deplete it. That doesn't mean you have to cut people out entirely (unless they're super toxic at which point you should). These might still be casual friends to have a laugh with now and then—a fun person to run into and catch up with over a cup of coffee. But give your energy to relationships that are reciprocated, to friends who show up and cheer you on.

Also, be true on your end, too. All relationships require effort on both sides. They are rarely an even 50/50 split (as life often gets in the way and sometimes one side has to give a little more), but just like you shouldn't expend energy chasing others, you also shouldn't expect others to chase you.

Authentically be present for the people you love. Show up for the people who have shown up for you. Your friend is in a play or has a big game tomorrow? Go cheer them on. Another is grieving a breakup? Go sit with them. Be there, in the sadness, and just let them know they're not alone. And don't be a fair weather friend. Don't be that person who chases the glittery sparkle of the popular crowd, leaving your real friends in the shadows, only to crawl back to them when that sparkle fades. Remember who your ride or dies are.

## 2. Reach down and lift others up

Remember how it felt when someone threw you a lifeline? Be that lifeline for others. I am here today, calling myself a published writer, in large part because so many other women and writers who have done it before me were willing to show me the way, warn me about potential pitfalls as I navigated the journey, and toss me a map when I needed it.

Whatever career field you're in, there will be opportunities to reach down to those coming up the ranks after you and give them your hand. Never forget how it felt when someone did that for you. And, never forget how it felt when someone didn't—and don't be that person. We're all better when we lift one another up.

And the same goes for motherhood and sisterhood. Don't be a gatekeeper. Have a life hack that makes everything easier? Share it with the struggling mom next to you—not in a *"I know everything"* kind of way, but instead, in a *"this helped me and I wanted to share it in case it can help you"* kind of way.

*This sound machine is a game changer! My kid is finally sleeping through the night.*

*OMG I am in love with my new breastfeeding bra—I'll send you the link if you want.*

*Hey, let me watch your kids this afternoon for a few hours so you can have some alone time.*

*I saw your kid melting down at the park. Mine is the same way these days. You're doing great.*

These are lifelines. Throw them out whenever you can and build a web of women and mothers who support one another.

## 3. Learn to forgive—including yourself

Make your choices about who you keep in your life, not necessarily based on whether they've messed up or hurt you (because, yes, we hurt the ones we love) but based on what they do next. Are they fighting for you? Are they doing the work to repair things? Showing you what you mean to them? Then they probably deserve a chance.

Also, forgiving someone who hurt you is a gift you give to yourself—not them. And stubbornly refusing to forgive just creates a ball of anger within you that grows and festers and corrodes your insides. Forgiving takes away the power that ball of anger has and, instead, releases it, leaving room inside you for joy and positivity.

Even if that person doesn't apologize, doesn't make it right, and doesn't seem to deserve your forgiveness, you're not doing it for them. You're doing it for you. If you're going to move on without them in your life, letting go of that ugly feeling of hate and anger is part of that process.

Even more importantly, learn to forgive yourself. You're going to make mistakes. You're going to hurt people you care about. It happens to all of us. Do the work—recognize your wrong, and make it right. Apologize (in a real, authentic way). Do better moving forward to prove that your apology meant something. And then forgive yourself. Because holding on to old pain and old regrets just allows that molten ball of negative energy to come back, take hold, and control you again.

### 4. Learn about yourself

I didn't start really learning about myself—about why I am the way I am, what causes my anxious thoughts, what makes me ultimately crash and burn—until well into adulthood. That means I lost so many valuable years when I could have been self-reflecting and learning coping strategies to help me live better. (I talk about this more in Chapter 13.)

Think about your best days and your worst days. What makes you feel immeasurably happy and completely filled up? What depletes you and causes you to be overwhelmed? What do you need to thrive?

It isn't always easy to learn truths about yourself because they don't always come in pretty packages. But everyone has something that makes their life harder and the best thing you can do for your own health and happiness is to name what exactly that thing is and take ownership of it.

### 5. Put goodness out into the world

This can mean so many things—it can be as simple as seeking joy and laughing as much as you can. Putting laughter out into the world means someone else might hear your laughter or see your joy and become infected with a little positivity.

It also means doing good and surrounding yourself with others who do good. You'll learn (if you haven't already) that some people are toxic and cloud the air around them with negativity. They may be coming from a place of pain, and we can still have empathy for that. But when you can identify someone who is simply hateful or someone who unfairly judges others, the best thing you can do is separate yourself. And then counter the bad with good. Think about a scale—how can you put goodness out there to blot out the ugly?

*Hold the door for the person behind you.*

*Be patient when an older person is walking slowly nearby.*

*Smile at a struggling mom and tell her she's doing a good job.*

*Tell the cashier her hair is beautiful.*

*Say please and thank you to everyone—even if they don't say it back.*

You'll feel lighter if you're good, and heavier and downtrodden if you're not.

### 6. "Choose your hard"

This common saying (attributed to Devon Brough) applies to most of life's choices.

*It's hard to stay in a toxic relationship, and it's hard to leave.*

*It's hard to be vulnerable and open up to new people, and it's hard to be alone.*

*It's hard to take care of yourself, cook healthy foods, exercise, and prioritize your mental health. All that takes work. But it's hard to wake up every day and feel terrible, too.*

*It's hard to put in the work and succeed at something. But it's hard to sit there and feel unfulfilled, watching your life pass you by, regretting that you never took a chance on yourself.*

*It's hard to fail. It's also hard to never win because you never tried.*

*It's hard to forgive. It's hard to not forgive.*

*It's hard to do the work and better yourself. It's hard to stay stuck where you are.*

*It's hard to take risks and put yourself out there. It's hard to look back on your life, regretting all the things you never did.*

*You'll have to pick your hard for the rest of your life.*

*As kids—do you try out for the team and risk not making it? Or not try and never know if you would have?*

*As teens—do you aim high for a college and career path that may not work out? Or play it safe?*

*As young adults—do you stick it out with the long distance relationship because you're in love? Or say goodbye and move on with a broken heart?*

There's not always a clear path of which choice is better for you. You might pick your hard and half way down the road realize that you need to turn back and go the opposite way after all.

But one thing remains constant: The journey may be hard, but the feeling of pride you'll feel as you look back and see that you gave it all you had—whether it works out or not—that's the good part. That's when you get to say "I did that. I tried really hard."

Because that's all we can do in life.

## Notes on Chapter 19

**This list isn't carved in stone.**

Remember that the life lessons you're teaching your kids are ever-evolving. This list fits my family, right now. My kids are 16, 14, and 12. I've had a lot of years to think about what matters most as I prepare them to launch into the world on their own someday.

# Lessons for My Kids (and for Myself) as We All Grow Up 133

(And as I prepare to launch myself into the world post-SAHM life.) This is not what my list looked like 10 years ago, and it will probably change as we all continue to grow up.

In the end, I'm pretty sure all of us just want our children to be good and kind and help the world be better, not worse. How to get them there? We'll figure it out along the way.

# Chapter 20

# The Death of Martyrdom

> **The 21st Century SAHM**
> @21stcenturysahm
>
> People are like "My mom never complained! She did it all with a smile, was never tired, never asked for help!"like somehow running ourselves into the ground while SMILING is a better alternative than speaking openly about our struggles & supporting one another.

**H**ave you noticed that martyrdom is dying?

One of the best things that younger generations of women have figured out is to stop this toxic game. Today's moms are realizing that sacrificing ourselves so we can wear our "*I do it all and never accept any help!*" badge isn't the life we want.

For generations, women were martyrs, in part because they didn't have a slew of alternative options. *Grow up, make babies, raise babies, cook dinner, clean the house, smile, look perfect, hide your pain.* (I think that was the list, right?)

In the past, women were not allowed to have careers, leave unhealthy or unsafe relationships, or seek alternative paths in life. Hell, they weren't even allowed to open their own bank accounts. Therefore, it's not surprising that they also didn't ask for help or talk openly about their struggles. It probably didn't even seem possible.

And I do think the need for martyrdom has carried over into motherhood today although it seems to be dying out. I can recall, back in the baby and toddler days, when I was committed to wearing my martyrdom crown. One time, my husband was gone for a particularly grueling work trip while I was elbow-deep in diapers and sippy cups. And I was so damn tired and overwhelmed and a mom-friend spotted it immediately on my face.

"*Let me watch the kids so you can get a break,*" she said.

And I said no.

She said yes.

I said "*No, really, I'm fine.*"

She insisted.

I finally relented and agreed to an hour or two, and she replied that nope, she was taking my kids for the entire day.

And this back and forth went on until yes, I agreed to actually practice some self-care and take a much-needed break. But why did I fight it so hard?

I think it was mostly the guilt. Generational martyrdom has ingrained the message into our brains that if we accept help (or, gasp, *actually ask for it*) then we're not good mothers.

Accepting help means we're weak, mothers are told.

It means we are failing.

And it means we aren't allowed to wear our coveted "*I do it all*" motherhood badge.

But what happens when that badge is hanging on a specter of a mother, barely there, ashen-faced and drowning? When the badge falls off anyway and rattles to the floor because there was nothing for it to hold onto?

Women and mothers are finally realizing that we'd rather be here, be full of color and strength and life, and let the martyrdom badge go out with the trash. But it has taken (at least for moms like me) a bit of a push to ask for help, accept the help, and finally still believe that we're doing a good job.

The fight to kill off martyrdom has also been met with some resistance, namely from those who have so tightly wrapped it up into their identities that they seem to actually *thrive* on self-sacrifice. Do you know women like this? Women and mothers so determined to martyr themselves that they'll pin that button directly onto their skin—they don't give a fuck. You cannot help them with the kids. Or the house. Cooking? *Get out of their kitchen.* Cleaning? *Nope, they got it.* You see them quietly sip coffee all day because they aren't allowed to get tired! *Sickness? Power through! The flu doesn't stop a woman on a mission to do it all by herself! What is rest? Rest is for shitty moms! Real mothers don't let near-death viruses bring them down.*

So, yes, whether it's lack of alternative options or the inability or unwillingness to release the toxic hold of martyrdom, women have been running themselves into the ground for, well, forever.

Today's moms though—they're changing the narrative.

Today's moms are saying, "*Welp! House is a mess, but I'm doing my best. People live here!*" And "*Nope, dinner isn't made even though I was home all day. Take out or PB&Js it is!*"

And, most importantly, they aren't letting moments like these reduce their worth or value as mothers.

Also, moms today are sitting. Can we all stop and appreciate the power of just sitting down? If I have a quiet minute during the day to do something for myself, do you know what I do? I freaking sit. I sit with a book or randomly scroll Instagram on my phone or flip on whatever is hot on Netflix and let my body REST. And I cannot express to you how damn good it feels to let go of the guilt. Because you can be 100 percent assured that if I'm sitting and resting, the house isn't clean. There's still laundry to be done. The sink is full of dishes. And I have a list of no less than 10 things I needed to get done this week like "schedule allergist appointment" and "refill the dog's medication."

The list is never complete. We never have everything done. But we're resting anyway.

Because, yes, if I have a quiet moment when no children are around to ask me to drive them somewhere or help them find something that is directly in front of their eyeballs or whine about how we have "no food" when we actually have chicken, cheese, bread, bananas, apples, cereal, milk, and around 9,000 other choices, I will take that moment for myself and simply rest in the peaceful quiet.

Martyrs don't sit. Martyrs don't rest. Do you understand how revolutionary it is to be a mother who sits? Our grandmothers sure never did that.

Your martyr membership is revoked if you take care of yourself—if you rest.

So, yeah, when I let that mom-friend help me that day, I lost my martyrdom badge. (Did I ever have one anyway though?)

Every time one of us sits and reads a book or sleeps in on a Saturday or leaves the kitchen a mess and grabs a drink with a girlfriend or asks our husband or partner to grab a pizza on their way home from work because we took the dog for a walk in the sunshine and listened to a podcast instead of cooking, we float farther and farther away from the stain of martyrdom.

Today's generation is changing the narrative. We're talking about how hard motherhood is. We're asking for help. We're accepting help. We're caring for ourselves so that we aren't ghost-like apparitions with the life drained out of us because we've given every drop to others, leaving nothing for ourselves.

And here's the best news of all: Letting go of our Club Martyrdom memberships does not mean we are weak. It actually means we're strong and self-aware.

Strength lies in facing the reality of motherhood. Doing it all without help isn't a life I want to live. It's isolating and exhausting and it means spending all my days and years chasing an impossible goal. And at the end, I'd be a pile of dust—my shroud falling to the floor as my loved ones say, *"Here lies Mother, who did everything for everyone and nothing for herself, ever."*

Hard pass.

Strength means realizing how much more vibrant and meaningful motherhood is if we're healthy. Today's mothers want to experience all the joyful but fleeting moments with their kids. They want to be there for the T-ball games and band concerts, and that might mean running to a weekend tournament and leaving behind a messy house and piles of laundry.

Strength means tagging in our partners to get the baby in the middle of the night because we need rest, as well. Neither of us have an easy day tomorrow and we'll want to be the engaged, present mom our kids deserve.

Personally, I thrive on strength and health and feeling powerful. And I will be none of those things if I am a martyr.

Today's women are telling the truth: Motherhood is hard. Harder than any of us thought. (It always has been.) And some might say we're whining. They might even say this book is whiny. But I say we're finally being honest, and I think our grandmothers would be damn proud of us.

## Notes on Chapter 20

***The takeaway here is blunt:***

Don't be a martyr. There's no prize. You won't win. Take care of yourself, sit once in a while, rest, ask for help, accept help, and honor our grandmothers, who didn't have a choice, by showing them that by showing them that we're figuring it out.

If you want to wear a motherhood badge, wear the one that says, "I take care of myself so I can be here, be present, and make memories with my family for a long time."

That's the real badge of honor.

## Chapter 21

# "Everything Is Fine," "I Don't Care What Other People Think," and Other Lies We Tell

**W**e lie a lot as women and mothers. I do it. You do it. Our mothers did it and their mothers did it. We do it in part for self-preservation. And we do it because telling ourselves these untruths is all we've ever known. These are the rules of motherhood we've been taught; rules that are ingrained into us.

Lying to ourselves doesn't mean we're failing this motherhood thing, but it's about time we finally call these statements out for what they are, don't you think?

Here are five lies we tell, whether we want to admit it or not.

## The Lies of Motherhood

### 1. Everything is fine

It's not, and that's okay.

I have three kids. Two are teens, and one's a tween. There is never a day when every single thing is fine. Ever. Just as the clouds part over one's struggles, another seems to step into their own storm. I move from kid to kid, holding up umbrellas, helping them navigate life, face disappointment, sadness, pain, rejection, stress, fear of failure, or even just their anger at me because I had to be a parent and say, *"No, you can't have Snapchat at 11 years old."*

And because moms carry it all (physically—the diaper bags, the toys, the snacks and drinks, and figuratively—our children's fears, stresses, losses, and heartache), we're not fine.

*We're not fine when our middle school daughters are mourning the loss of a bestie who has moved on.*

*We're not fine when our kids aren't invited to a birthday party and everyone else at the lunch table was.*

*We're not fine when our kids measure their self-worth by a number on the scale or what they see in the mirror. (And we're not fine when we do it either.)*

*We're not fine when our body temperature soars 20° on a random Tuesday and we pit out through our clothes in the chips aisle while our kid talks back, saying you "never let him get anything fun" because he wants a $7 bag of habanero chips and you look with rage at your overflowing cart full of meats, fruits, cereals, ice creams, and, yes, chips that are less expensive and less likely to sear off his inner stomach lining. Because OMG you try so freaking hard and nothing you do ever seems to be enough to make everyone happy.*

So, no, we're not fine.

And that's okay.

Because life is too much of a constant shit-storm for us to be fine. But that doesn't mean we're quitting. We'll plow through, head-first, into the shit-nado, everyday, dodging a bullet here—*"Everyone has a phone except me! My life is ruined!"* and another one there—*"Mom, you have a weird hair growing out of your chin,"* pit-stains and all.

We're not fine, but we're still here. Now be a dear and get us some ice water, would you? Or maybe just put us in a quiet freezer somewhere for a few hours where no one can tell us we're horrible mothers because we won't buy our children $120 leggings or because we wouldn't let our kid eat Skittles for breakfast.

**2. I don't care what _____ thinks**

I don't know a single woman or mother who doesn't care what other people think. But if you're out there and you have actually mastered this craft, please share your wisdom with the rest of us. Because we all say it. And we all want to believe it in ourselves.

*I don't care what Becky from the PTO thinks.*
*I don't care what my ex thinks.*
*I don't care what ____ (close family member, neighbor, or even distant relative you only see on holidays) thinks.*

But we do care. We let their dumb, pointless opinions get to us. And it's infuriating. Because allowing someone else's opinion, especially when they often don't know the truth of our lives, seep into our psyche only diminishes our self-worth.

Caring what the mean mom at school pick-up thinks as she side-eyes your messy car or clearance Walmart sweats doesn't serve you in any way. She has an opinion of everyone, and none of them are positive. But that's a reflection of her own insecurities. Judging others just highlights Mean Mom's low self-esteem even if her fancy car is immaculate and her sweats are designer-brand.

Your ex? Whether it's an ex-spouse, ex-lover, or even ex-friend, remember, there's a reason they have ex-ited out of your life. It's better for you that way, so ex-it their opinions out of your mind too, because they don't matter. I know, I know, easier said than done, but if you find yourself allowing an opinion of an ex to impact your well-being, practice mindfulness. Close your eyes, visually imagine removing this thought from your mind, and replace that empty space with a positive thought about yourself—like how funny you are. How much your kids love you. How good you are at your job. How you have a new, loving partner who appreciates you. How you have girlfriends, ride-or-die besties, who are 1,000× times better to give your time and energy to. Find something that's true (and positive) to fill that void so that you no longer give credence to your ex's opinion (because it doesn't matter).

Do you have a toxic family member or neighbor or really anyone else in your life who loves to spew opinions about you? Like how you parent wrong, you dress wrong, your house isn't clean enough, your kids aren't _____ enough (insert words like "*well-behaved*" or "*athletic*"), or you're too _____ ("*loud,*" "*opinionated*")?

Treat them like they are the school bully from middle school. First of all, their opinion is irrelevant. But even though you know that, their comments can still get to you—I know, I've been there.

But this is how we respond to bullies. I tell my kids that when someone insults or teases them about what they look like, for example, to respond with, "*Well, I like it!*" Boom. Insult shut down. When someone says, "*Your hairstyle is dumb*" and you respond with "*I like it,*" that jerk has nowhere to go, so they'll move on.

The same goes for crotchety old Aunt Mary who lectures you because your kids wear jeans to church. Or your super-opinionated organic neighbor who thinks you're a bad mom because you give your kids popsicles with food dye.

"*We're fine with what we wear to church!*"

"*We're fine with popsicles in our house!*"

At this point, all they can do is repeat themselves, which they might. But you've decided their opinion doesn't matter and that you're a good mom, even if your kids *eat popsicles in jeans on the way to church*. (You're still a good mom. And Jesus loves you and your kids, regardless of what Aunt Mary says.)

Same goes for opinions about your messy house or loud laugh or whether you wear too much makeup or not enough makeup or your clothes are too tight or too baggy …

"*I like it!*"

That's it.

### 3. I've got this

You might not actually. I love the sentiment, and it often helps when we're facing a big life challenge to tell ourselves this mantra. I encourage my kids to say it when facing something huge—*"Believe in yourself! You've got this!"* I'll say, as my son heads out onto the ice to play the hockey game of his life, as my daughter trots off into line, ready to perform in a horse show, or as my oldest faces a tough math test he's been studying for all week.

But the truth is, sometimes we simply don't have it, and that's a tough reality to accept. Sometimes, my kid flops out on the ice and just doesn't bring his A-game. Sometimes, my daughter scores last in a horse show because the competition was just too fierce that day. And, sometimes, my math-whiz kid doesn't shine as bright as he had hoped he would on those geometry proofs.

They said to themselves, *"I've got this,"* but turns out, they didn't.

And the same thing happens to us, as women and mothers.

We, of course, tell ourselves this positive statement, and we have every intention of handling whatever it is. But sometimes, the universe has other plans.

Years ago, I can remember pushing a full cart through the grocery store. My very defiant two-year-old was in it, the four and six-year-old were skipping alongside me, asking 831 questions and touching everything. We were almost at the end of the shopping trip when the little one asked for something and I had said "no"—his least favorite word.

That's when, in response, that little stinker opened an egg carton and threw an egg on the ground. Of course, everyone looked. Of course, judgy eyes sent me the *"you need to discipline that child"* glare. I wanted to cry. I wanted to run away from my life in that moment. But I had still had to pay for all of the food in the cart, take those three kids home, and be a mom.

I did not, in fact, *"have this."*

When I gave every drop of energy and patience I had throughout the 2020–2021 school year to get that same stubborn toddler (who by then was a second grader) through virtual school, bribing him with candy, Fortnite skins, whatever it took to get him to pick up a freaking pencil and *please just write a sentence for the love of God*, and I finally gave up one day and said something like, "Fine! Whatever! I don't care if you go to school anymore!" (I don't remember exactly—it's a blur) and then felt like a piece of old crusty dog poop immediately after because he was eight and was not meant to attend school on a screen and it wasn't his fault and he missed his friends and teacher.

I did not "*have this*" that day (or any of the other days during that grueling first year of the pandemic).

But did anyone "*have this*" in 2020? Did anyone weather that storm with complete and total grace?

Haven't mothers everywhere also faced the challenge of buying groceries mid-toddler meltdown?

Because that's the thing to remember. We might tell ourselves this lie: "*I've got this.*" And we might 1,000 percent believe we do, but when we don't, that doesn't mean we're failures. It means we're regular women, regular moms, walking head-first into the hurricane called motherhood every day, sometimes watching in horror as an egg falls on the floor, sometimes losing our cool during a pandemic, but never giving up.

We just go back in and try again.

### 4. I can't show weakness, sadness, grief, etc., in front of my kids

As moms, we often feel that we have to be strong all the time. We shouldn't let our children carry our pain or our burdens. We should shield them, protect them, keep them innocent, keep their world magical. We don't want them to look back and remember seeing their mom break.

Angelina Jolie once shared in an interview that while going through her divorce with Brad Pitt, she'd only cry in the shower so her kids wouldn't see or hear her. I understand why she did it that way, but here's the truth about motherhood.

They already know, whether we try to hide it or not.

Sure, our children may not hear us sob in the shower, but they see our red eyes when we get out.

They see our hunched shoulders. They notice we're quieter than usual. They pick up on our lack of patience, our short tempers. They see how tired we are and how the color has drained from our faces.

I do think there is value in protecting our children from pain and hurt if we can. That's one of the most important parts of our job.

But we can't shield them from it all. And we can't always hide every moment of weakness or emotion we have either.

Grief is a part of life, and if your kids haven't experienced it yet, they will. And it doesn't just accompany death. Grief happens when a friendship ends. Or a boyfriend says goodbye. Or a career path doesn't work out. Or when motherhood doesn't look like you thought it would because you face infertility or your child has unexpected medical needs. Or when you move to a new state and say "*See you again someday*" to old neighbors who watched your kids grow up. (I talk more about motherhood grief in Chapter 24.)

At some point, our kids will face heartbreaking scenarios like these if they haven't already.

So, if Mom is feeling sad, it's normal and healthy to share that information with your kids so that they know it's okay for them to sometimes feel sad too.

This idea that we as mothers have to be rock-solid steel and never break in front of our kids is, to me, unrealistic and yet another unattainable ideal that sets us up for failure.

Then guess what feeling like a failure does? Makes us even more upset.

And round and round we go.

Instead, if we allow ourselves to show, in front of our children, that we're human, that we sometimes feel sad or angry or disappointed, then we aren't perching ourselves on the top of a fragile, unstable pedestal that likely won't hold us up anyway.

But most importantly, we are paving the way for our children to also have emotion. Life is going to knock them down, just as it's knocking us down when we're crying in the shower. And maybe when they're having a bad day as adults, they'll feel comfortable calling us so we can be there for them. Because they'll know it's okay if mothers sometimes break.

**5. *The kids' needs always have to come first***

Actually, the parents need to come first. Because what happens if we're not here?

Last weekend, my husband and I handed the kids a long list of chores and pretty much peeled out of the driveway for a day date. First stop was Home Depot (as one does after 20 years of marriage) to look at plants for the yard. On the way back, we hit some smaller local nurseries, too, and realized we were hungry.

Several hours later, we were paying the bill after enjoying a huge plate of nachos and a couple beers. We spent the time not only talking about where to plant boxwoods and hydrangeas but also sharing dream vacation destinations and when we might renovate our old, dated kitchen. And how we'll downsize some day after the kids are gone and move into a cute lake house with a boat by the dock.

It ended up being exactly the day we needed, and it didn't involve our kids at all.

Obviously, sneaking away for the day was easier for us as our children are older and don't need babysitters anymore, but we've prioritized ourselves and our marriage since they were babies. We sneak away at least once a year—for a local weekend hiking in the fall or, if money allows, a bigger trip to a beach resort where we day-drink cocktails in infinity pools instead of refereeing who gets the last Oreo.

We are extremely fortunate to have grandparents who can swoop in and handle the circus that is our lives when we're gone, and I know not everyone has that option.

But prioritizing our marriage doesn't only include trips. There are nights the kids might hear us say, *"Eat something remotely healthy for dinner, watch a movie, and put yourselves to bed at some point. Mom and Dad are off duty."* And we pour ourselves a drink, sit on the back patio, and have ourselves a little date night.

Because listen, our children are loved and safe, and we provide endless joyful core memories for them. But part of the stability we provide comes from us nurturing ourselves and our relationship.

Marriage is a plant that needs to be watered. It needs to be fed. And it needs lots of sunlight. And anyone who's been a parent for more than five minutes knows how easy it is to neglect it. You get too tired to water it. You don't have time to feed it. And you're so busy giving your kids all the sunshine that your own adult lives can be forgotten in the shadows.

The same thing goes for self-care for both of us. We both work really freaking hard at life. Whether it's motherhood or fatherhood or careers or taking care of our home or making sure our parents are okay, there's a lot. And we sometimes forget to rest. We sometimes have to remind ourselves to stop, eat a vegetable, drink some water, and get some sleep, even if that means saying *"No, Mom can't do \_\_\_\_"* or *"Dad can't be there for \_\_\_\_"* to our kids. Because we want to keep being there for as much as we can for a long time. We want to host Christmas for our grandkids someday and steal them away for the weekend so that our kids, who will be exhausted from the crashing waves of parenthood, can take time to nurture themselves.

But all that only happens if we're still here. If we still like each other. If we've taken care of ourselves so that we have enough energy and joints that move and hearts that beat.

Our marriage and our own well-being is the base of the pyramid—the foundation. We need to keep it strong and stable so the 8,000 daily needs of our three children can rest upon us. And that's not to say that stability requires a two-parent household. Or that a couple should stay together no matter what. There are a myriad of reasons why it's better for the entire family unit if the relationship ends and the kids have a more solid, secure foundation that way.

In our house, we've learned over the past two decades that this marriage is strong and worth fighting for, but it needs water. I need water. He needs water. We both need sunshine. And to be the kind of parents we want to be (and the kind of parents our kids deserve), we have to make sure we aren't forgotten in the shadows.

And sometimes water and sunshine looks like a day date to Home Depot followed by a couple beers and a plate of nachos.

## Notes on Chapter 21

*We all lie.*

It's true. And sometimes lies serve a purpose. Saying to yourself, "I've got this" is a good exercise and helpful in a million scenarios.

Just don't forget to forgive yourself if you don't "have this." And if everything isn't "fine." If your kids saw you break down. If you let Mean Mom's judgmental comment get under your skin.

Let yourself have a bad day, and let your kids see you, on occasion, have a bad day. Then pick yourself up and sneak out for a day date, even if it involves looking at hydrangeas that are on sale. The kids will be alright.

# Chapter 22

# How I "Lost Myself" but Found the Pieces and Put Myself Back Together

It sounds so cliché: "*I 'lost' myself in motherhood*"—but damn if it isn't true. At least, it was for me. I was shrinking, almost like I was a character in *Avengers: Infinity War*, feeling my arms, then legs, then torso, then head slowly turn to sand and disappear.

Everything I knew about myself to be true suddenly felt gone. I was smart (*gone*). I was good at my job (*gone*). I was important (*gone*).

I didn't know it was happening—the shrinking—but that's the thing about motherhood. You don't really have the mental space to do a whole lot of self-reflection when you're moving through your days in a zombie-like trance, tasked with keeping a tiny blob of mushy skin, spit-up, and weird green poop alive, even though you yourself feel like a mushy blob as well.

But it did happen. I lost myself. I lost all sense of self-assurance. I lost all sense of competency. I felt small and dumb and, frankly, invisible. As if I'd turned to dust and floated away.

However, the one good thing about losing yourself is finding the lost pieces along the way and slowly putting yourself back together. Like one of those wooden nesting dolls we had as kids—first the tiny piece in the very center, then another layer as the top and bottom snap together, then another, and another. Like the pieces of a puzzle, each one fitting back where it goes, until you are whole again.

As I contemplate this next step on the journey of life—what I'm going to be and do when the kids are grown—I'm not entirely sure the pieces are all back yet. I might still have a few loose ends, a few extra layers to add, but I'm close.

And I can look back now at the past 16 years of my life as a SAHM and accept that, although I did lose many parts of myself in motherhood, there were a few distinct times I found myself again along the way.

## Meeting Sabrina

You know how there are moments in life, people you meet, that you're 1,000 percent sure saved you? Well, joining a SAHM playgroup was one of those life events for me. I had just moved to Kansas as a new mom and, disappointingly, did not find a slew of other SAHMs to have coffee with and share breastfeeding stories with in my neighborhood. Thankfully, it was 2009 and the internet was there to bail me out.

I found a meetup group that frequented indoor play areas and even hosted playdates at moms' homes if they felt inclined to open up their front door. After a few months, I'd attended a few meetups, made small talk with fellow SAHMs, and it was good. It was able to break up our long days, have adult (although interrupted) conversations, and have a reason to shower and put on real clothes. But so far, I hadn't really clicked with any of the moms in the way

I'd hoped. They were all nice, but I could tell that no one was going to be my new bestie, which I so desperately wanted.

Then, one day, we hit an indoor toddler climbing gym and I spotted someone I hadn't seen before. Her back was to me, and I could see that she had a baby in a carrier on her chest and bright blonde hair.

Something in my mind said, "*There she is. Your new best friend.*"

And she was. Sabrina (name changed for privacy) and I could not be more different. Her blonde hair stood in stark contrast to my brown. Her baby was tiny and fit snugly into a carrier. I never bothered with those as all my babies came out the size of toddlers. She was quiet and never yelled at her kids. EVER. I morphed into Khaleesi in the *Game of Thrones* finale when my kids refused to put their shoes on.

Despite our differences though, something organic was there. Pretty soon we started doing babysitting exchanges. She took my toddler and baby some days, I took her toddler and baby other days, which meant each of us got a quiet day to ourselves! BLISS.

But honestly, I think one of the best things about Sabrina was the feeling I got when I walked into her house. It looked like a family lived there. A family of four that included one baby, one toddler, a mom, and a dad.

Up until this point, I was still operating under the "*I'm a failure if my house isn't clean*" rule. And I definitely, DEFINITELY would never have a friend over if it wasn't scrubbed top to bottom. That meant hosting playdates (which I desperately needed) but also hours upon hours of work cleaning beforehand (and cleaning after).

But when I walked into Sabrina's house for the first time, there were toys on the floor, dishes in the sink, and dust bunnies in the corners. And she didn't say anything. She didn't apologize for the mess. She welcomed us in, and that was that.

And let me tell you—it felt like a literal BALM on my soul. I didn't know we could do that! I didn't know we could just have people over and let our houses look like they normally looked. I didn't know a friendship could feel like this, in motherhood.

My friendship with Sabrina was one vital piece of putting myself back together.

## Running the SAHM Meetup Group

I've talked quite a bit in this book about how my teaching years were such a pivotal time in my adult life. And how abruptly walking away from my career caused unexpected grief that I wasn't sure how to process. I know now that saying goodbye to teaching was particularly hard because I no longer had a leadership role.

*"How can you say that? You were a mother—a Mama Duck, with all her baby ducks in a row!"* you might respond. And yes, I was now a Mama Duck, but the leadership opportunities provided in a professional setting are far different than the ones that exist at home, in a toddler playroom. Thankfully, this was a void in my life soon to be filled.

After a few years of attending events with the meetup group that saved my life, the previous "head mom in charge" who handled things like organizing events and monitoring requests to join was stepping down. And they needed a new leader.

Here was another puzzle piece.

I offered to take a shot at holding the reins, and damn did it feel good. The feeling of importance, the feeling of almost having a ... job? Even if it didn't pay, I had responsibilities! We had meetings! MEETINGS.

With over 70 members throughout our community, we'd often meet to discuss new ideas for activities, address any drama going on in the group, and ensure that everyone was respecting the rules (like what to do if your kid bit another kid, things like that).

Sometimes, those meetings were at night at a coffee shop without kids, which meant I got to go out. OUT! In the evenings! For a MEETING. Do you know what that does for a former professional with a master's degree who used to wear ironed pants and now just dreams of washing the spit-up out of her hair?

I could literally feel myself rejuvenating.

## Writing

One day, I wrote a humorous Facebook post about taking my toddler and newborn to the grocery store and my family and friends loved it and encouraged me to keep writing. (I wrote about this more in Chapter 16.)

Having dreamt of being a writer since childhood (a dream that, it seems, got a bit derailed), something came alive that day. An old passion resurfaced—the dust blew off—and I thought, "Okay, yeah. Maybe I'll start a blog. Maybe I'll write again."

Only a few people ever read the blog; it just didn't take off. But what did happen was I started submitting my work to other parenting sites. And after a few tries, they started saying yes.

Before long, I was freelancing and writing for *Scary Mommy*, *Babble*, *The Huffington Post*, *Her View From Home*, *Motherly*, *Sammiches and Psych Meds*, and any other online publication I could find. If you were perusing online parenting articles anytime between 2012 and 2020, you may have come across something I wrote. Allergies, potty-training, SAHM-life, work-from-home life, politics, the pandemic, I wrote about it all. I was hustling my ass off and never said no to an assignment.

And I saw my name in print. For years, I wrote articles for *KC Parent*—a free parenting magazine often found around town at local businesses. This meant I could grab food to cook for dinner and see an article I wrote on my way out of Hyvee or Pick and Save (our local grocery stores). Also, my work was selected to appear in a few anthologies about parenthood, which meant I had real books in my hand with my name in them. REAL BOOKS.

I was making a little money for the first time in years, but more importantly, editors were telling me that they wanted my words.

MY words. And I could feel that empty cup, that need to feel smart and important, filling up again.

I had found another layer that had been lost years ago.

## Speaking Opportunities and Conferences

As my social media following grew and as my publications piled up, I started getting messages from people wanting to work with me. ME! Karen Johnson, at home, in 10-year-old sweats, typing away on an old dinosaur laptop.

*You want ME to come speak at your event?! You want ME to wear a real bra and blow dry my hair and look like an actual human lady who goes out into the world and talks to people?*

But it was true. I spoke at a Baby Expo and a Saturday morning meetup group for young moms. I prepared speeches, showed up in a blazer and cute boots with a heel, and watched as people sat there and listened to what I had to say.

I got on airplanes—AIRPLANES! And flew to conferences in other states where I'd connect and network (a word I'd never used in my life) with other writers and content creators who were big on social media. I sat in sessions, learning how to hone my craft, and I made new friends and colleagues—COLLEAGUES! I had "work friends" again. Work friends to go to dinner with, room in hotels with, and brainstorm ideas with.

More life was breathed into the ghost of old me as I reclaimed an identity other than Mom.

## The Popsicle Post

In 2017, I went mega-viral. I wrote a post (known by lots of people as the "popsicle post") in which I talked about the many, many ways to be a good mom. Here's an excerpt:

*"Are stay-at-home moms better than working moms? NO.*
*Are working moms better than stay-at-home moms? NO.*
*Are married moms better than single moms? NO.*
*Are you a better mom if you take your kids on exotic vacations? NO.*
*Can you be a good mom if you the closest thing you get to a vacation is the park? YES.*
*Can you be a good mom and have a super scheduled summer with lots of planned activities? Yep.*
*What about if your summer is lazy with no plans? Yep.*
*Do good moms let their kids watch TV? Yes.*
*Play video games? Yes.*
*What about if you say no? Also fine. Your choice. You're the mom. And a good one."*

Well, the post clearly resonated with the world because it ended up being shared 579,000 times and I gained 100,000 new followers in 24 hours. If you don't speak social media, that's a whopper of a viral post (especially for 2017 when Facebook was the big show—remember, this was pre-TikTok and Instagram was still a baby).

Even our local news network reached out to interview me! I actually drove downtown to be ON THE NEWS because of this viral post. It was surreal and a big moment for me. I had written something so impactful that it touched every corner of the country and was spreading around the world as well.

Important? Valuable? Smart? Influential? Yeah, I was finally feeling all those things again, and boy did it feel good.

## This Book

This book surely won't be the final piece (because are we ever done building ourselves?) but it's a big one. Perhaps the final, outer layer of the wooden nesting doll, ready to be put back on the shelf for display. Then a new puzzle to start. The next phase of me—the phase that will carry me into the "post-kid-at-home years"—because they're coming, whether I'm ready or not.

Like Sally from *The Nightmare Before Christmas*, all of these events have felt like me sewing my parts back on, piece by piece, and now I'm beginning to feel whole again.

---

## Notes on Chapter 22

*You're still there.*

I know you feel lost. Like pieces of you are missing. But listen, they're still there—all of them. They might be scattered about. You might have to search extra hard for a few. But keep going. Keep looking for that mom-friend you organically click with, or an opportunity to exercise your brain muscle and make you feel smart again, or a challenge that reminds you how capable you are.

It might seem overwhelming to get on a plane and leave your kids for a professional opportunity or a chance to see an old friend you've been missing. But you'll probably really, really love it once you get there and you'll come home full of life and inspiration and a newfound appreciation for all of the many things you are—other than Mom.

You're there, I promise. You haven't turned to sand, even if it feels like you have. And it's time to rebuild.

# Chapter 23

# How Did I Get Here? (The Story of Our Gladiator Turtles, Medically Fragile Dog, and One Dead Plant)

Being the default parent means finding yourself in some precarious, often sticky (literally and figuratively) situations. It means that if an adult in your household is trying to catch vomit with their bare hands, it's probably you. Or if someone is cutting a poop-filled onesie off of a smiling infant who just blew up their world (and yours), it's likely you. And it also means that between you and your spouse or partner, the one driving around with a sick turtle in a plastic Tupperware container, yeah, that's you too.

Hmmm that's oddly specific, so let me back up and provide context.

I was in the middle of the 40-minute drive, heading home from the "exotic pets" vet. In the passenger seat beside me sat one of our aquatic turtles in a small container, along with a box of tiny needles and medication we'd have to inject into his little papery legs for the next 30 days that had just cost me $200. He was fighting an infection that the "exotic pets" vet attributed to "stress" after getting into a fight with our other turtle and having part of his face bitten off.

All of this is true. (Like I could make that shit up.)

And it was at that moment, glancing over at 200 bucks worth of doll-house sized injectable needles that I said out loud, *"How the hell did I get here? What even is my life?"* (The turtle didn't respond.)

## The First Turtle

Okay, I'll back up even further. 2020 brought a lot of change to many households, ours included. We became what many referred to as a "lockdown house." Because one of our kids has a scary health history with asthma, and the fact that both my husband and I were able to work exclusively from home, combined with the school offering virtual instruction for a year, we decided to hunker down and wait the pandemic out a bit until we knew more about it.

That meant no playdates, no activities, no get-togethers with family, and no vacations. What it did mean was loooooots of free time. And my middle child (who was nine at the time) seized this opportunity, beginning a long, arduous, and ultimately successful campaign to become the owner of a pet turtle.

My first response to her asking, *"Can I get a turtle?"* was *"No."* (And many, many responses after remained in the negative.) Absolutely not. I am not a reptile fan and had no interest in owning a pet that eats bugs and can't be snuggled.

But she was not to be deterred and, with the extra hours of time in her life to fill, began researching all that was involved in turtle care—proving to me, eventually, that she was very serious about this endeavor and would undoubtedly be a responsible owner of an aquatic turtle. So, as one of our first adventures out of the house that year, we headed to the pet store in November 2020 and brought home Pumpa, a razorback musk turtle.

Pumpa was a challenge from day one. He was very antisocial and hid all day long. He did give us one scare and embark upon a brief (and terrifying) hunger strike that also required a trip to the "exotic pets" veterinarian when he was only a few weeks old. After dropping him off (they had to keep him for observation because of course they did), my daughter asked how he seemed in the car. *"Well, sweetie, he didn't say much,"* I replied. After some medication and whatever else vets do for tiny starving antisocial baby turtles, Pumpa thankfully started eating again and didn't die. But he still hid all day long and didn't climb on any of the many (many) trees, rocks, and basking platforms we'd invested in, so my daughter suggested we give him a friend.

## The Second Turtle

In May 2021, we added Bjorn, a map turtle, to the tank, hoping to "bring Pumpa out of his shell" (ba-dump). This experiment would turn out to be an epic fail because sometimes friendships just don't work out (see Chapter 10). Bjorn was very outgoing and wanted to play, while Pumpa did not. And for the first few months, Pumpa did everything he could to avoid Bjorn's prodding. But, we later learned, he was apparently also plotting his revenge.

One day, we came home to a bloodbath. It was like Fight Club in there, and Bjorn, the little one, definitely didn't win. Not only was part of his face missing, but he began to show other signs of infection and needed some medical intervention. That's when the second 40-minute drive to the "exotic pets" vet occurred. (Did you know that you can't just roll up to a regular vet with a reptile? I didn't. I do now though.)

## The Dog

Also in 2021 we got a dog—because why not? The pandemic really did us in folks. Wrigley is a lovable and uber-friendly Bernedoodle. He's like the Bjorn of the dog-world. He's in your face, does not believe in boundaries, and would probably get his face bitten off by another anti-social grumpy dog or cat or other household pet because he doesn't read the room.

However, he is plagued with heart-breaking violent seizures and is, therefore, on a whole bunch of medicine twice a day, for life.

## And the Plant

As our lives returned to normal and we re-entered the world in 2021, we, of course, got busier and busier again. Also, our kids are older and can (and should) handle more responsibilities around the house, right? RIGHT.

So, I put my daughter, age 10 at the time, in charge of our one indoor plant. It was a Spath Peace Lily—a huge, hearty, very hard-to-kill plant, and we loved it so. But by this point, I was in the eye of the storm, trying to save one turtle from being Gladiator-ized by another turtle and living in fear of another traumatizing seizure for our 80-lb dog. (Plus, there were those three kids I was running after, too.)

I told my daughter that keeping that plant alive was her job. A plant we'd nearly killed at least 10 times, and every time it simply refused to die; it always rejuvenated when we'd remember it was there and water it.

Reader, the Spath Peace Lily sadly passed on. It was apparently a plant of 10 lives, not 11. And out to the trash it one day went.

## No More Living Things

And that's the day I told my family that I was officially at capacity. I was not going to care for another living thing. We were not getting a replacement plant. We were not getting another pet. And we were definitely not growing any more humans in my uterus.

Three kids, two parents, two violent turtles, one epileptic dog, and one dead plant.

That's our pandemic story and (most of us) lived to tell the tale, for which we're grateful. The turtles were separated by a wall for a while that they constantly tried to knock down because they apparently had a death wish, so eventually we had to invest in an entire second tank and another filter, UV light, and a slew of additional fake plants and rocks as well. The turtles are never getting back together. Like ever.

The dog is still hyper and joyful and stealing everyone's food. We've gone from two pills a day to eight, but finally seem to have the seizures mostly under control.

And the planter is empty. And empty it shall stay until someone else in this house wants to be in charge of refereeing turtle fights or driving all over town for expensive pet medications. Or, at the very least, watering a damn plant.

How did I get here? No idea. But being the pet mom and plant mom are apparently other jobs that are just handed to us because who else is going to put the starving and/or mangled turtle in Tupperware and drive it to the vet? No one, that's who.

---

## Notes on Chapter 23

*Do not keep reading if you're hoping for actual advice.*

Being the default parent means also being the primary pet parent, apparently. It means being the only one who remembers to administer daily (life-saving!) dog meds. It means being in charge of watering the plants or doling out that task to another human who will likely forget. It means driving tiny baby turtles to the vet in the middle of the day and then driving them back home.

It just does. Default parenting isn't just managing the kids. It means managing the household and everything in it.

Our high-maintenance dog has to get groomed every eight weeks. Who schedules that and takes him to and from the groomer? Who do you think?

He had a tick on his ear recently, so he needed a blood test to rule out Lyme's Disease (which was thankfully negative) but yep, that was me, too. And when he ate a grape, when he was randomly limping for a few days, and when he was due for vaccines? Me, me, and, oh yeah, me as well.

Running low on dog food? *Adds to cart.*

Turtle tank dirty? *Finds time in schedule to clean it (with daughter's help!).*

The default parent is the CEO. It's up to you whether you want to pass some of that off to other people. I tried with the plant (it didn't end well). If you have the magic formula and you can get other people in your household to remember to brush your bernedoodle so he doesn't have to get shaved and look like a circus dog, please share the secret.

Because, as I discussed in Chapter 6, even if I pass off tasks like giving Wrigley his medication, I still worry that whoever is now in charge will forget, and I will hound, text, call, send in a homing pigeon to make sure it gets done. Therefore, to quiet my worry, I just end up doing it myself.

My advice here is to do better than I am doing. Put these responsibilities on other people. Actually, for real.

Then tell me how you did it.

# Chapter 24

# The Many Forms of Motherhood Grief

Grief comes in many forms. There's the bring-you-to-your-knees grief that takes over when someone you love dies. And if it's motherhood grief, that someone you're mourning could be your own child, which is a level of grief and pain that trumps all others.

But as mothers, we feel loss, pain, heartbreak, and disappointment in other ways as well. That's because motherhood grief takes on many forms.

Motherhood grief sometimes comes in big, tsunami-sized waves, and other times in smaller, less overwhelming, but still painful moments that feel like cracks in our heart.

Women and mothers in all corners of the world grieve as they endure infertility and pregnancy loss. There's no way to prepare for that tidal wave crash, and it can feel lonely, isolating, and block out all the joy and sunlight for a long time.

Grief also happens when children have terrifying health scares or life-long medical conditions that might mean they have a drastically different childhood than other kids. And usually that means their parents' lives also look very different from the lives of other moms and dads they know.

Mothers grieve when our children grow up, and we have to bid farewell to those precious baby days when our little ones fit in the crook of our arms. When those quiet middle-of-the-night feedings are over and although we're thrilled to sleep again in more than three-hour chunks, we already miss that bonding time when it was just us and our baby in the twilight hours.

We grieve when the toddler phase has passed, and we suddenly have school-aged children who can actually do quite a bit on their own. When we have to drop them off at that first emotional day of kindergarten and realize that from this day forward, the world will get a lot more of our child's time and focus and we might have to stand in the background for the first time after we've been the center of their world all these years.

Then, years later, the teen years hit. Oh is there grief in raising teens. How is it possible to miss someone so much who is right down the hall? But we do. We miss them already because they're starting to break away from us. And because we know what's coming next.

And then the next part happens. And the grief that a mother feels when her child drives away, heading off toward their own new life. There are no words. I haven't had to do it yet, but I've sat with friends who have and grieved with them. I cried all summer long before my oldest entered high school, suddenly feeling like my time with him was very fleeting, so I have little hope of actually keeping it together when my kids fly away from our nest. (My therapist will be very busy—this much I know.)

But tiny moments of grief are sprinkled in too, especially when we realize we've hit another "last" and have to cope without warning that we'll never again carry our sleepy child to bed or read them a story at night or rock them to sleep. When all of a sudden they say, "I can walk into school by myself, Mom" or "I already ate dinner when I was out with friends" or they simply say goodnight and "It's okay, Mom. You don't have to tuck me in."

We grieve when our children grieve. When they lose a friend, are hurt by cruel words, or feel left out or don't get on the team, or aren't accepted into their dream college. We feel ourselves crack inside and break into pieces as we wish we could scoop up their pain and hold it for them until it passes.

We grieve when we walk away from careers that we love so we can stay home with our babies. Whether by choice or by necessity, there is still a mourning that occurs within us as we bid farewell to the person we once were and the life we once lived. That's real grief, and we should acknowledge it so mothers can process it better, heal, and know that they are still good moms even if they miss their old selves.

And we grieve when motherhood doesn't turn out like we thought it would. I know I sure did.

This is one type of grief I was not prepared for. And one that has, at times, brought me to my knees with sadness. The truth is I couldn't always give my kids the mom I wanted to give them—the mom they deserved—when they were little. And I had to spend some time grieving this.

The times I yelled, the times my overwhelm got the best of me, the times I was touched out, the times the noise became too unbearable, the times they saw an ugly, angry face on me that they didn't deserve because they were just being children. All of it happened, and all of it has caused me grief and regret.

So, what do I do with my motherhood grief? What do any of us do? We sit in it for a bit, and when we're ready, we get out of the pool, dry off, and start to heal. Because even if you grieve parts of your motherhood story, when you take a step back and look at the whole picture, what do you see? Think of your motherhood years as a quilt, patch by patch added with each new experience. Sure, maybe there are some frayed sections here and there, but look at it. All of it. It's a masterpiece—one that you'll hand down to your children, as you teach them that they, too, are allowed to be imperfect and are allowed to grieve when life gets hard. And then they can wrap themselves in the quilt you made and know that they'll be okay because their mom taught them how to heal and forgive themselves as well.

## Notes on Chapter 24

*Grief is a part of life.*
No one gets to enjoy all their years on this planet without experiencing the darkness of grief, sadness, regret, and then hopefully, healing in the end. Motherhood, particularly, can be chockfull of grief, which is really a kick in the teeth at times because we give this job everything we have.

Knowing it's coming your way (if it hasn't already), here are three ways to cope when motherhood grief has sucked the air out of your lungs:

**1. Don't fight it.**

Honestly, one of the best things you can do when you're caught in an avalanche of grief is to just sit in it. Fighting it will take all your energy, and you probably won't win. You won't be stuck in the snow (or ocean, or whatever metaphor works best for you) forever. But if you're grieving your child growing up and moving away, spend a day crying big fat tears, sitting in a sea of baby pictures, and let it out. It's okay—healthy even—to cry and feel sadness. These are normal human emotions and suppressing them will only cause them to feel heavier on your soul.

You won't sit in the pool of grief forever. Eventually, you'll feel that the despair has poured out of you and you'll be ready to get up and go outside again.

**2. Take care of yourself.**

Grief is powerful and can take away all your strength, leaving you barely able to keep your eyes open and get through the day. Self-care at this point doesn't have to be huge. It can be as simple as remembering to drink water and taking your dog for a 10-minute walk (maybe tomorrow you'll be ready for 20). This is also a good time to say "Yes, thank you," when someone offers to cook you a meal, take your kids for an afternoon, or help you with chores around the house. A bit of self-care will help you regain your old self.

**3. Talk about it.**

When someone has lost a loved one, usually the best way to cope with grief is to talk about the person who died. Whether it be a spouse, a parent, or even a child. Saying their name and keeping their memory alive is an essential part of healing. The same goes for other types of grief. If you're grieving the end of a motherhood chapter like the last time you breastfed, or you're about to send your firstborn off to kindergarten (or college!), find solace in connecting with other moms sitting in the same grief. Or moms who have been where you are and are already on the other side of healing—they can show you the way.

But don't bury it. Don't hold it in. Every mother grieves at some point. You're not alone and you are strong, even if the tears keep coming.

# Chapter 25

# Always Awkward, Never Cool

How does that old prayer go? You know the one—asking God for help to change the things you can, accept the things you can't, and the wisdom to know the difference or something like that.

As I've mentioned before, I believe there is great power in learning about yourself. I didn't really begin active self-reflection until well into adulthood, but holy smokes did light bulbs go on when I did. And I think the reason this prayer is so widely used is because it encourages us to always better ourselves and change the things about us that we can change. But it also helps us realize that there are just some personality traits that stick, and it's a fruitless endeavor to fight them.

For me, that fruitless endeavor is trying to be cool. (Or as my middle schooler would say, "sigma.")

Looking back, I've been a little awkward my entire life. Sure, I doodled the names of my crushes in my diary, teased my hair, and lip-synced to Paula Abdul and Madonna just like the other girls.

But did the other girls also write novels and bind them with twine at eight years old? Did they also get anxiety-induced migraines, stressing about being perfect in third grade? Did they wear their jeans backward in middle school because it looked like a fun idea? Or make a tie-skirt (thank you, Mayim Bialik, aka Blossom, for the inspo)? Maybe, but I doubt it.

When I look back at my childhood and adolescence, the evidence is there. I wasn't without friends. And I wasn't too far outside the "cool kids" circle. Usually, I hovered right on the bridge between cool and nerd and even made my way all the way across a few times to get invited to a party here and there.

But my visits to "cool kid island" were brief, and I ended up back where I belonged, in my comfortable spot where I got good grades, stayed out of trouble, and listened to Disney movie soundtracks while the popular kids were jamming out to Nirvana.

The truth is, I felt out of place in that circle as I was, and always will be, a little awkward. A little weird, a little too loud, and never really, actually cool.

Today, as a mom in her 40s, I am grateful to have girlfriends who accept me for me. They know what they're getting, and they invite me anyway.

They're getting a woman who at any given time will unexpectedly choke on water (sometimes air) and make an embarrassing scene.

They're getting a woman who doesn't know how to stand cute for pictures. A woman who must have missed the class where they teach you where to put your arms and how to do the one-leg bend in group pics. Last time I tried that, I bent my right leg too far and it disappeared from the picture entirely so it looks like I had a limb amputated.

They're getting a friend who falls a lot and walks into door frames because she's lost in her head and not paying attention.

They're getting an ugly crier. Like blotchy, swollen eyes, excessively boogery, the whole bit. So inviting me to a sad movie for Girls Night Out? A bit of a gamble there.

They're getting an awkward runner. I didn't know this until I participated in a family fun run with my kids at their school a couple years ago. My husband snapped a pic of me as I came around the corner (on mile ONE), and I was already overheated and showing signs of pain in my face.

They're getting someone who is usually three to five years late to fashion trends, home design trends and, well, just trends.

Also, they're getting a friend who apparently doesn't know how to fix her face when recorded. I attended a Packers game with some friends a year ago, and because I'm super lucky, one of my closest girlfriends has front-row seats. FRONT ROW. (SHE is actually cool.) We ended up on TV, not just during the game, but on replay for a while as highlights were shown in the days after. The girlfriends I was with: They they understood the assignment. Their cheering faces were happy—faces of joy! And there was me, with a strained smile, looking stressed out, and maybe like I had to poop. Of course, I wouldn't be me if I had pulled off looking cute (instead of constipated) on NATIONAL TELEVISION.

So, yes, when they choose me, my friends are getting a girlfriend who is almost always awkward, no matter the circumstance.

But guess what else they're getting?

*A friend who is funny.*

*A friend who is a talented writer.*

*A friend who is hard-working and passionate about what she believes in.*

*A friend who will be there to celebrate their wins and hold their hands in grief.*

*And a friend who is a good mom.*

Because while I have learned, looking back at my four decades of awkwardness, that I have never and will never be "cool," I have also realized that I have some pretty great qualities—traits I can see I've passed on to my kids. Traits that are maybe even better than being the "cool kid" after all.

So, as we near the end of our SAHM or #momlife era and think about what we're going to do and who we're going to be next, I think it's important to reflect on what we've learned about ourselves (or get going on that self-reflection if you haven't yet!).

What are the truths of who you are? What personality traits are you most proud of?

As we stand on our front porch, waving goodbye as our last child drives away, and we, in that moment, step into some new shoes, let's not hide. Let's not shy away from the "real" us, whether we're nerdy or cool, loud or quiet, introverted or extroverted.

We can always work to better ourselves, but we should also face the truth of who we are at our core.

I'll go first. I am a book-lover. I love musicals and comfy clothes and quiet time at home. I like structure and predictability and using a paper wall calendar even though it's 2025. I don't wear makeup more than once a month, and I fluctuate between uber-pale and semi-pale throughout the year. I've had the same brown boots for 10 years, which has worked out great because they've come back into style three times. I fall asleep watching *Friends* every night and someone from my family usually puts me to bed like I'm a child (or a grandma).

I love to laugh, drink wine (and beer), and travel the world.

That's just who I am and I've decided that, rather than spending a lifetime trying to be cool, I'm instead going to learn to like myself and embrace the real me. Why pretend to be something you're not? Especially when what you actually are is pretty great, too, just in an awkward-where-do-I-put-my-arms-when-I-take-a-picture kind of way.

You can spend your life trying to be somebody else, or you can accept that you might choke on water at dinner and spit it on your husband's coworker.

Either way, you have a lot of good stuff to put out into the world. And what's cooler than that?

## Notes on Chapter 25

*Hi! Are you awkward too?*

If you're struggling with accepting (and even loving) your awkward self, let me share with you something I've told my kids. My daughter once described a popular "mean girl" to me, saying "Ugh, she'll probably be a model or something someday."

"Yeah, she probably won't," I replied.

Because, if you think about it, usually the "cool," popular kids—especially if they're mean—those kids peak in high school. And that's it for their glory days. When you reconnect on social media 10 years later or show up at your 20-year class reunion, that popular boy or girl that blew you off or even bullied you when you were kids ... they're just a boring old regular person now. Likely in a stagnant career, semi-miserable, still clinging desperately to the glory days of high school.

But you know who's doing great? Awkward you. Awkward me. The regular kids. The kind kids. The kids who never saw the top of the pedestal in high school, so they had nowhere to fall from.

I tell my own children this all the time. Just be authentically you, be kind, be a good friend. And the rest will fall into place. It's okay if you don't know how to stand in pictures or if you look constipated on national TV at a Packers game when you're in your 40s. Because you know what? You're going to have a ball that day with your girlfriends who love you for you.

# Chapter 26

# Halfway There (and Livin' on a Prayer)

**W**elp, here we are, friends. Middle aged. Remember how *old* "middle-aged" people used to be? And now it's us. I'm 44. If I'm lucky enough to live a long life, I'm officially halfway to 88. Half of my life is behind me, the other half in front. And the years that are left, well, they aren't the younger years, that's for sure.

If you, like me, are not young but not old, if you still stay up late partying once in a while but you need eye glasses in the laundry room now to read the instructions on clothing tags, that might mean you're around halfway there, too. So, let's stand together at the top of this mountain and take in the view.

We've spent 40-something years hiking up to this summit, and hopefully will spend another 40+-something on the descent. But as we stand here, at this peak in our lives, let's take a look at the lives we've built—the *legacy* we've built. We've done the work, we've given every drop we had, and we're far from done.

When you stand there, at the midpoint of your life, the side of the mountain you climbed up on your left, the path down on your right, what do you see? Is it beautiful? Breathtaking? Is it lush and vibrant or do you see barren patches across the landscape?

I'll be honest. My view isn't 100 percent what I want it to be. Sure, there's a lot of beautiful scenery out there and I'm damn proud of everything I've accomplished so far, but the land out there needs some water, too.

Because when we look out at the landscape of our lives and see those patches of lifeless desert, I think they signify things like this:

- Guilt
- Self-loathing or self-doubt
- Criticizing ourselves because we're too loud or talk too much or we're too quiet and don't assert ourselves enough
- Berating ourselves because we have fat on our stomachs or cellulite on our thighs or wrinkles on our faces
- All the unkind things we say to ourselves that we'd never say to our kids or girlfriends or anyone else we love

This is it, friends. This is the pinnacle atop the mountain, and we owe it to ourselves to see all the beauty we've created. But that requires us to see the beauty in ourselves.

To appreciate the view in front of us, in order to water those dry patches of land that makeup the lives we've lived and the lives we're going to keep living, we need to make a few changes and work on ourselves a bit.

Here's what I'm working on to make my view a little bit healthier and prettier:

## Two Important Ways I'm Working on Me

### 1. I'm dressing my body in a way that makes me feel good

I don't know about you, but I've noticed that although the clothing industry is changing for the better and becoming inclusive of more body types, still, more often than not, the models don't look like me. I see an outfit I like, order it, and then don't like it. Hmmm maybe it's because in the ad, the model was a size two. I am not.

And because I loathe in-person shopping with every fiber of my being and would rather pour hot wax into my eyeballs than try on 841 items in a dimly lit dressing room only to find that one or two of them work, I do as much shopping as possible online, from the comfort of my home. That also means I've spent a lot of time in the last few years seeking out online shops whose models look like me now, not me at 25. Seeing a bathing suit or tank top or shorts or pair of jeans on a 40-something mom with cellulite and belly fat is empowering as fuck I've realized, and that's the type of shopping culture I want to be a part of. It also gives me a better mental image of what the item will actually look like *on my body* once it's delivered.

I also purge anything that doesn't fit in my closet. Gone are the days of holding onto something that doesn't fit anymore even if I really, really love it. Even if it's the dress I wore to one of the most memorable events of my life. The memory is still there, the joy I felt wearing it remains in my heart and mind. But staring at something in my closet that no longer serves me, that no longer makes me feel beautiful and instead highlights my insecurities—that's the type of thing that blocks that breathtaking view we're all seeking.

Jeans too tight? Bye. Get new jeans. That's it. Immediately gone.

And the same goes for my kids, especially my teenage daughter, whose body is also changing at a rapid pace lately.

*"Mom, all of my pants are too small,"* she said to me one day.

And we went shopping that afternoon for new pants, to fit her new size—whatever it was—then filled a donation bag with everything that didn't.

Also, I'm all about comfort. If I'm usually a medium, but the large fits better, I get the large. Whatever. So the tag says L instead of M. Neither of those letters really say anything about me as a person. But if I'm uncomfortable, I'm grumpy, and that DOES say something about me as a person.

And I chose styles that allow me to move with confidence. If flowy shirts make me feel pretty and at ease because that means I can eat and drink and enjoy myself, flowy shirts it is! I don't need to wear clingy fabrics or fashion trends that don't make me feel good. Hard pass.

**2. I've changed why I work out**

I work out regularly and I work out hard—I always have. I sweat buckets, I get that "good sore" in my hamstrings and abs and triceps, and I push myself as hard as I physically can.

And my body doesn't change, whether it's Pilates or weight lifting or straight cardio. I know because I've done them all, over and over. Weeks go by. Months go by. Years go by. And my body is ... well, it's stubbornly settled into what it's going to be at this stage of life.

Now I have a choice. I can:

A. Quit working out because what's the point? If I don't *"lose weight"* or *"get smaller,"* I'm failing, right? That's what the world tells us!
- Or -
B. Change my reasons for being down in my basement, dripping with sweat and saying four-letter words to someone who says I need to hold that plank for another 15 seconds.

I choose B.

Imagine if society empowered women by instilling in them these benefits of exercise and healthy eating:

- Living a long life so we can chase our grandkids around someday
- Having strong bones so we can fight osteoporosis
- Maintaining good heart and lung health so we have energy to travel and see the world
- Helping to prevent or heal from joint pain, muscle pain, nerve pain, or any other random ailments we wake up with now that we're middle-aged

- Improving our mental health and fighting feelings of anxiety and depression, which are common among women our age
- Creating a sense of community among women as they cheer each other on and work toward new fitness goals
- Encouraging women to believe in themselves that we can do hard things! We're badasses!

Instead of:

- Making ourselves smaller

Imagine how empowering that would be.

Listen girlfriends, I'm not getting smaller. I might get more toned here and there and turn some stubborn fat into muscle (or I might not). But I've been around the same weight for a few years now through all the various fitness routines I've tried. Also, I'm not giving up my favorite foods unless I medically have to. That means I might have a chicken salad on a Tuesday for dinner, but if my kid's team wins a tournament and we're all out celebrating, I'm absolutely going to have a beer and a bacon cheeseburger that weekend and feel zero guilt about it.

Also, I will never give up chips because salty snacks are life and that's a non-negotiable.

We deserve to soak in the beauty of this view atop this mountain. We've given a hell of a lot to get here, but it's on us to choose what we see.

It's on us to water the plants and feed the animals out there and, well, nurture it.

*Nurture us.*

It's on us to look in the mirror and be kind to the person looking back at us.

To toss jeans that don't fit and remind ourselves that a number on a tag doesn't define our worth.

And to look out at the horizon and see the life we've built and feel nothing but pride in all that we've done.

As we stand at this midpoint, some might say *"It's all downhill from here,"* which is fine. We're ready and strong and we promise to enjoy the descent (even if we need to put on our reading glasses to clearly see the directions).

Because as the great Bon Jovi told us when we were kids, we might be halfway there, but if we hold hands and do it together, we'll make it—I swear.

---

## Notes on Chapter 25

***Some tips to help you achieve these changes in mindset:***
Buying clothes is expensive! Simply purging clothes that don't fit and going shopping isn't feasible for lots of people, but hanging on to stuff that makes you dislike yourself is damaging to your mental health. So, here are some things to try:

- Clean out your closet and sell items on Facebook Marketplace, at a garage sale, or consignment, then treat yourself to something new with your earnings!
- Shop consignment yourself. Someone someone else is probably doing the same closet purge you are. Plus, you did something good for the earth by repurposing items.
- Join local "buy nothing" groups in your community. People are always giving away items that could work for you. And this is where you can donate your no-longer-needed clothes to someone else. Everyone wins!

On changing your "reasons" for exercise and healthy eating:

- Set new fitness goals that aren't weight- or size-related. (Mine have included doing 20 pushups in a row, running a race, holding a three-minute plank, completing an advanced level fitness program, lifting the next heaviest weight, etc.)
- Focus on the sense of pride and accomplishment you feel as you get stronger and take better care of yourself. Let that feeling wash away the toxic pressures of trying to make yourself

smaller. (I weigh more than I did 10–15 years ago, but I'm 10× stronger, so that's a win for me.)
- Join a fitness group—in person or online. My accountability group has been together for over a decade! We don't all live near each other, so it's just a Facebook group where we check in and share our fitness goals, successes, and struggles and cheer each other on. Or meet up with girlfriends to walk, run, or hit a class together. You'll love getting stronger and healthier if you do it with your besties.

# Chapter 27

# Make Me a Promise

> "I don't think you should ever have to apologize for your excitement. Just because something's cliché [that] doesn't mean it's not awesome. The worst kind of person is someone who makes someone feel bad, dumb, or stupid for being excited about something."
>
> —*Taylor Swift*

There's a lot we can't control in life, like aging and getting turkey necks and when our three-year-olds poop in the pool and our teens give us that blank *"you don't know anything"* stare even though we've lived on this planet three decades longer than they have. But we do get to be the boss of a lot of things, one of those is doing the things that make us happy.

And I'm telling you—nobody deserves to do something that makes her happy more than a hardworking mom. But, sometimes, it takes us a while. We're programmed to give every drop of lifeblood that we have to our families (see Chapter 20 on martyrdom). Our lives become so busy that it's hard to fathom those cute suggestions people make like *"Take time for yourself!"* and *"Don't forget about Mom!"* (I know, because I say them, too.)

But something happens when we hit our 40s, doesn't it? I think it's called *"not giving a fuck."* And damn it is refreshing. That doesn't mean we stop caring about kindness or we aren't bothered if we hurt someone. That stuff still matters. I'm talking about doing what we want, liking what we want, and wearing what we want. I'm talking about forgetting those stupid rules we grew up with that dictate how we live and curb our joy and life experiences. Rules that actually don't matter, like *"Don't wear white after Labor Day!"* (Seriously? Why is this a rule? Who actually cares?) Or those sexist, oppressive rules that women can't wear short skirts after age 30 or bikinis at the pool with their kids.

So, to those of you out there reading this, please make me a promise. (Better yet, make yourself a promise.) Promise to do the things that make you happy even if some archaic societal rule says you shouldn't because you're too old or because you're a woman or because it's October.

Here are eight things that make me immeasurably happy and I don't care who knows it:

## My Unapologetic Happiness List

### 1. *Christmas music starting November 1*

I get it, *"Don't forget about Thanksgiving!"* people. I hear you, I do. Personally, I don't really care about Thanksgiving. I don't like turkey, and I'm meh on mashed potatoes. I'll eat an entire apple pie like the apocalypse is coming though, so it's not like I don't appreciate what Thanksgiving has to offer. (And the family time is pretty great, too, of course.)

But I don't have an emotional attachment to Thanksgiving and personally don't care even a teeny bit if it's overshadowed by Christmas. Christmas brings me a feeling of joyful nostalgia passed down from generations of women who loved it as much as I do, so I cherish it and I want to extend the season as long as I can. One month of holiday magic isn't enough, so for me, it starts on November 1 and I make zero apologies for it. (Also, in the same category is this admission: I love alllllll the holiday music—yes, including Mariah Carey—and sing it loud and proud. I said what I said.)

### 2. Musicals, taylor swift, and '90s hip-hop

I'm writing this book at the height of the Eras Tour/Travis Kelce insanity and I. Am. Obsessed. I love this story, I love her, I love the Kelces. I lived in Kansas City for nine years and will forever love the Chiefs, so this merging of worlds is, well, it's just beautiful to me and it makes me happy, and no, I do not care if you think I'm too old for this investment. Obviously, I don't know what the future holds for these two lovebirds, but right now, it's a happy thing. I'm also completely intoxicated with *The Tortured Poets Department* and have become a bigger Swiftie than my teenage daughter. Again, I make no apologies. I have listened to *TTPD* for approximately 9,000 hours and love it more and more every time. Female Rage Taylor is exactly what this perimenopausal mom needed as it turns out.

Also, '90s hip-hop. Is there anything better? I read once that we always love the music we listened to during our most formative teen years—and, well, it's true for me. Snoop, Dr. Dre, TLC. These jams make me think of those care-free nights of driving around town, hoping to run into my crush or my bestie's crush (no one had cell phones back then, so we didn't know where anyone was). When I'm grumpy and have to clean the house against my will, blasting a little Warren G or Salt-N-Pepa instantly changes my mood. I love '90s hip-hop and make zero apologies. (Also, if you get me to a karaoke bar, I will immediately forget that I have negative talent and I WILL attempt to rap "Slim Shady.")

Finally, musicals. I grew up on stage and am now raising a thespian as well. We have great appreciation for musical theater so listening to *Hamilton, Six, Hadestown, Moulin Rouge,* or even the soundtracks to *Aladdin, Moana,* or *The Little Mermaid.* All of this is very likely to go down in my house or car at any given time. Get on board or find another ride.

### 3. My own comfort

If I don't wear another piece of clingy fabric again for the rest of my days, I will have reached the pinnacle of life goals. Because honestly, I'm done. I'm done feeling like my clothes are too tight. I'm done feeling self-conscious because I have full intentions of eating and enjoying life in whatever I'm wearing, and that means wearing clothes that provide room for growth.

I also loathe being too hot or too cold. Obviously, some of that is unavoidable. For example, my kid plays hockey, so I'll freeze in a hockey rink every weekend watching him play without hesitation. And I'll swelter in the hot sun watching another child play tennis and cheering on my daughter at horseback riding competitions and supporting my baseball player in the summer months. I'm there for all of it.

But if I'm sitting through a 90-degree baseball tournament, I'm wearing a tank top and shorts and not giving that a second thought. Here are my legs, world! They've got cellulite and spider veins! I'm not covering up as boob sweat pools into my bra and I melt into a puddle on the sidelines of a Little League game. Not doing it. If that means the world can see my back fat, so be it.

### 4. Taking naps

I went through all of the baby and toddler years without resting. And if I did, the guilt overwhelmed me so I didn't enjoy it or reap the benefits of this form of self-care. But a few years ago, I found myself just simply exhausted from life, probably, and I started taking occasional naps.

Have you ever done this?! Naps are glorious! I had no idea. The idea of just simply lying down for an hour and closing my eyes even though the kitchen was a mess, the kids were out of clean socks, and there was no dinner plan, it seemed impossible. Until my perimenopausal body said "enough" and just quit on me. Until I was left with no choice but to just listen to it, take a nap, and wake up rested and ready to get back to the list.

Now I don't hesitate to nap if my body is saying it needs one—even though the voices in my mind occasionally still try their guilt trip "*Good moms don't rest*" story (see Chapter 20 on the death of martyrdom). The good thing about naps is that you stop hearing those voices when you're sleeping.

### *5. Salty snacks*

I am 100% aware that a good reason my body probably doesn't change, despite working out often is because of my diet.

Of course, I try to eat a healthy diet (I really do feel better after some leafy greens!) but you will have to pry my Doritos, honey mustard pretzels (Dots are the best!), or Chex Mix from my cold dead hands. I will eat salty snacks late at night until I die or until a doctor tells me I'm about to die if I don't stop. I do not care. Crunchy snacks at night, after all of my jobs are done and I'm finally taking some time for myself to veg out and watch *Friends* reruns (see #6 on this list), make me happy. The end.

### *6. Friends reruns*

I have seen every single episode of *Friends* enough times that I can pretty much recite them all word for word. But I have never (and probably will never) get tired of this show as it remains a pivotal part my nightly routine unless my husband and I are engrossed in a show like *Ted Lasso* or *Game of Thrones*. All the other nights ... it's me, my salty snacks, and that unrealistic purple NYC apartment that no one could ever afford in their 20s.

Like '90s hip-hop and Disney movie soundtracks, there's a comfort for me in watching old *Friends* reruns. It's me-time and I cherish it. I love every episode (although the trivia game, Ross getting stuck in leather pants, Ross at the tanning salon, and "See? He's her lobster!" are probably my faves).

Everyone who knows me knows how much I love *Friends,* and I make zero apologies for it.

### 7. *Books that make me feel things*

As a writer, a former English teacher, and an avid reader since preschool, I'm a book snob. I'll admit it. I don't always love the "hit" series or popular author everyone else is talking about. I love historical fiction. I love books that make me cry. Books that make me rage. Books with long-winded complicated sentences that have powerful female characters who inspire me to believe in myself—that I, too, can be strong and brave.

That means while everyone else is reading the latest bestseller that's getting made into a movie, I might be holed up in my recliner, sobbing over a story about a mom and her kids surviving the Dust Bowl on boiled onion soup.

I think people should like what they like and read what they want to read and not feel like they have to fit into some trendy mold. That's not what reading is about.

### 8. *Sticky-sweet internet content*

The internet can be a terrible, toxic, evil place. But it can also be a source of healing—a soothing balm on the wounded soul (if you tailor your news feed a bit.)

One of my favorite forms of self-care, especially through the tumultuous dumpster fire that has consumed news cycles for the last decade, is binge-watching an endless loop of cute, happy, emotional videos. Puppy videos—the best. The 22 hat moment at Taylor Swift concerts—I watch them all on TikTok. Footage of kids befriending the elderly or of soldiers coming home? Ack! My heart. LOVE.

Honestly, the world has seemed relatively apocalyptic for so long now that I think we all need reminders of positivity, kindness, and just sheer joy. If I need a real break from it all, escaping everything and watching 79 consecutive clips of dogs running into leaf piles or seeing their owners for the first time in months, yep, that's just what I'm going to do.

That's my list. Whatever is on yours, own it and be loud and proud about it. Hold on to the things that make you happy with a death grip and apologize to no one.

---

## Notes on Chapter 27

*What does your list look like? What are those simple things that you can (and should) enjoy even if society says you shouldn't?*

Want to binge-watch Hallmark movies where everyone wears plaid and falls in love in a gazebo? Do it.

Want to leave up Halloween decorations year-round because they bring you joy? Leave them up.

Want to wear a crop top even though you're 42? Wear it proudly.

Want to blast '90s hip-hop and eat popsicles on your back patio this summer? Crank it.

Promise me.

Promise yourself.

Like what you want to like, no matter what your age is or what your body type is or what time of year it is or whether other people tell you it's dumb.

No one gets to tell you what makes you happy.

# Chapter 28

# I'm a Total Fraud (by the Way)

I've spent a good chunk of this book telling you things like *"Believe in yourself!"* And *"Love your body!"* And *"Stop chasing perfectionism because it's unattainable and leads you down a road of exhaustion and disappointment!"*

But the truth is I'm a total fraud. Because I often don't believe in myself. I often don't love my body. And I haven't yet shaken off that fake cloak of perfectionism I've been carrying my whole life.

Even as I write this book, the one you're reading right now, I'm scared shitless. Scared no one will read it. Or scared people will read it—and what that means.

But I guess when I say the words out loud (or type them) it means at least I'm trying, right? Because the truth is I'm very much talking to myself when I preach about *"not comparing yourself to others!"* and say things like *"Your value isn't determined by a number on the scale or the tag on your jeans!"*

I'm just not not fully there yet.

I'm still on the side of self-doubt and haven't fully crossed over to a place of full confidence and self-assurance. (Does anyone actually ever get 100 percent there?)

I just want to be honest and call myself out for where I really am on this journey. Who I am, today, as I try to figure out what on earth I'm going to do when the kids grow up.

*I am a person who struggles with self-doubt.*

*I am a person who struggles with body acceptance and positivity.*

*I am a person who struggles to believe in herself and who sees the teeniest, tiniest crumb of not-success as utter throw-me-in-the-pit failure.*

*I am a mom who says platitudes to her kids like "If you don't believe in yourself, how can you expect other people to believe in you?" and then cowers in the corner, afraid to believe in my own self.*

I'm afraid of writing this book because what if everyone doesn't love it? (And I know that's nuts. There's no book everyone loves. "*Even Taylor Swift has haters,*" I'll whisper to myself as I peek, timidly, at my Amazon reviews.)

I'm afraid of telling all these vulnerable stories about how I haven't always loved motherhood (the world will brand me a shitty mom) or how I have resented my husband's success (that must make me a shitty wife) or how the SAHM baby and toddler days damn-near killed me (why am I not more grateful for those years?)

But then I think, okay, well I better tell the truth. And maybe these stories will help another mom whose doctor is side-eyeing her weight gain or a mom who has dreams she's too scared to chase for fear that the world will laugh at her or call her whiny and unappreciative of the life she already has.

Or maybe this book will just make another mom laugh as she notices that she, too, suddenly has a turkey neck and says, "Fuck it" and pours a beer.

But if I've ever seemed, despite all my "*Know your worth!*" campaigns, that I, actually, completely, know my own worth, I'm sorry to have deceived you because I'm not fully there yet.

I question my value. I allow diet culture and beauty culture to permeate my brain and make me say unkind things to myself. I berate myself when I make mistakes or say something dumb at a social event or look like a frumpy mom next to the trendy, super fit mom at school events.

And then I start writing. I start talking to you (and to myself) and we get a little better. We take another stone off of that path to perfectionism and add one to the real road we're on, where we have wrinkles and gray hairs and fat rolls but also joy and laughter and we get to eat cake.

We realize that we might never fully get there—to a place of complete self-assurance. A place where we simply just unapologetically like ourselves. But dammit we're going to try.

So, call me a liar or a fraud, but please stay here with me as we keep talking it out. The journey will be hell of a lot more fun if we have girlfriends alongside us, won't it?

---

## Notes on Chapter 28

*Don't give up.*

Remember the chapter about the water challenge? Our success lies in the fact that we're out here, doing it. Fighting diet culture. Fighting society telling us we aren't supposed to age. Doing better for our kids. Showing our girls that their real worth isn't numbers-based even if that negative self-talk still lingers inside us.

This book is honest. I'm still a work in progress, and I still have bad days of self-doubt. But damn it, I wrote a book! What are you going to do to continue to break that mold and prove that you're someone to believe in? What are you going to do today (and tomorrow, and the next day) to make sure you keep moving those stones off that path of perfectionism and self-doubt and instead, build a better road in front of you? A road that's heading to a place where women get to look like women who are actually 44 and who appreciate how badass they really are?

It's okay if you're not there yet. Or even if you never get there. Just keep drinking water and don't give up. I promise I won't either.

# Chapter 29

# We Can Do Hard Things (and Let Me Tell You How I Know)

Okay, I know thinking about next steps can be scary. What will you do when the kids grow up? What will you be? Will you put yourself out there and try something new? Will you dust off that degree and return to the career you worked hard for in your early 20s? Will you start over on a new path? Will you try entrepreneurship and go it alone as a business owner?

These options all might sound a little daunting—I get it. I'm right there with you. But here's one thing I know about women and moms: We can do hard things (a quote made famous by the beautiful and inspirational Glennon Doyle). We really can. How do I know?[1] Because we're already doing them, all the time, every day. Since the beginning.

Hi, you over there who grew a human inside your womb and pushed them out or had them surgically removed from you—yes, you! That's a hard thing—being literally ripped apart and sewn

---
[1] https://wecandohardthingspodcast.com/

back together like one of these fabric dolls we played with as little kids. But you did it.

Then you had to share that baby with the world and expose them to germs and mean people and pollution and creepy strangers at the grocery store. But you had no choice. You had to do hard things because you're a mom now.

- If you have ever gotten up four times during the night to tend to a teething baby who just wanted to comfort feed and be in Mommy's arms and then got up at 6 a.m. with a toddler who demanded your energy and attention for the next 14 hours straight, then you can do hard things!
- Ever dealt with a blowout diaper, the kind where your baby poops up their back and it's in their neck rolls and you're like *"How in the world was all of this inside your little stomach?!"* And then cleaned that all up in a public bathroom with a squirmy, slimy, poop-covered baby on one of the questionably unsanitary changing tables that folds out of the wall while your toddler crawled around on the disgusting bathroom floor and peeped under the doors at other people? Then you can absolutely do hard things.
- If you have held down your tiny child while doctors poked painful needles into their little thighs, knowing that life-saving medicine was important but feeling your heart shatter while they wailed with pain, you've already done one of the hardest things ever.
- Or taken a baby and/or toddler or a combination of both out, anywhere, in public. That's hard. Just literally leaving the house while being in charge of tiny humans and keeping track of them and not letting them run into traffic—that's insurmountably difficult. Deciding to put one of those cute little leashes on them and knowing you'll be judged (but knowing you'll also be judged if your three-year-old, who is a runner, takes off and ends up swimming with the otters at the zoo)—those are hard things, all of them.

# We Can Do Hard Things (and Let Me Tell You How I Know)   199

Or how about if you have:

- Hauled a thrashing kid out of a public place under your arm like a football ...
- Taught a small, stubborn child to relieve their body of poop and pee into an actual toilet and not their diaper, their underpants, the carpet, the couch, or the plant at church ...
- Taken a toddler to a public bathroom while you (heaven forbid) actually took the time to pee and watched in horror as they scurried their way over to the door, threatening maniacally to open it so the whole world can see Mom with her pants down. Or worse, lived through them following through on that threat ...
- Fought with a strong-willed child who either (1) straight-legged themselves and refused to bend, which meant getting them into the car seat caused you to drip with sweat and say lots of "grownup" words? or (2) noodled themselves, refusing to stand or walk but also refused to sit in the stroller ...
- Done the "letters puzzle" your kid was obsessed with or watched *Frozen* for the 9,000th time while thinking to yourself, "*If I have to see that puzzle or hear 'Let It Go' one more time, I'm going to throw myself into a black hole,*" but you still kept doing it, the 9,001st time, for them ...

Then you can 100 percent absolutely do hard things.

- If you've watched with agony as your tiny kindergartener (who was just seemingly born last week and is now old enough to wear their own Spiderman backpack) say "*Bye, Mom!*" and skip off into a colorful classroom, searching for the desk that has their name on it, oh you've endured one of life's greatest heartbreaks. Did you cross your arms and hold onto yourself tightly because it took everything you had to not run in there and hold them one more time? Then did you eventually turn around and walk out of the building, leaving your whole heart there in that little chair? Do you know how incredibly hard that is? And you did it.

- Have you felt your kids' childhoods rush by in a blur? Have you watched as that same little kindergartener, who is suddenly now taller than you, start to pack up their room, labeling boxes "clothes" and "books" as they get ready to leave for college? And there you are again, arms folded, desperate to hold on but knowing you can't, knowing you have to let them go as they once again say, "*Bye, Mom.*" Do you realize how much strength you have?

Or if you have:

- Dropped your child off anywhere where they'll have to be brave without you (while you'll have to be brave by walking away) ...
- Taken care of a kid with the stomach flu and tried to catch vomit. Or worse, have you been the one who is sick but everyone still needs you to get up and function ...
- Taught a nervous child how to ride a bike, promising "you got them" and then having to help them up when they fall ...
- Sat with your broken-hearted teen whose friends ghosted them ...
- Comforted your kid when everyone was invited to the birthday party but them ...
- Held the pieces of your child's broken heart ...
- Watched your child hurt or suffer through pain or illness, praying to God to let you carry the pain instead ...
- Navigated when to hover and help and when to back off and let them figure it out. And messed up sometimes, hovering too much or not enough, but just kept going ...

- Stood by your teen as they faced consequences for a poor decision ...
- Had to say "no" to your kid even though you wanted to say yes, but you knew they were getting too entitled. Or had to say "yes" because they deserved to hear "yes" but you were dog-tired and didn't know how you'd come up with the energy or the money ...
- Worked on finding that balance between teaching your children to stand up for themselves and take no shit but also be kind and empathetic to others' struggles ...
- Sat up with your teen, talking late into the night when you could barely keep your eyes open, but you did it anyway because OMG they're talking to you ...
- Gone without so your kids can have what they need ...
- Realized that parenthood was sucking the life out of your marriage and your own sense of self, so you clawed your way back to the surface before you and your partner both drowned and lost it all ...
- Cried in the shower because you didn't know WTF you were doing or how you were going to get through the day, but you eventually turned the water off, got dressed and did it anyway ...
- Endured the crushing, breath-sucking grief of pregnancy loss or infertility ...
- Worked at a whole other job while being a mom ...
- Gave up your career to be home with your kids ...
- Fought through the loneliness and isolation of motherhood ...
- Did your very best even if sometimes your best still meant feeling like a failure ...

Then you can do this next thing, too. Even if it's hard. Even if it's scary and you're not sure of yourself. You've been doing hard things for years—every single day, all day.

Stop doubting yourself, and start believing in yourself. There's nothing a mom can't do. Just look at all she's already doing.

---

## Notes on Chapter 29

*"I can do hard things."*

Write that down on a Post-it and stick it to your mirror. Whisper it to yourself as you're driving or working out or folding laundry or breastfeeding at 3 a.m.

And if you ever doubt it, look back on this list and count how many things you can check off. Now do you see it? You can do this next hard thing too.

## Chapter 30

# So, What AM I Going to Be When They Grow Up?

**F**uck if I know, but I do know this (TLDR):

I'm in my mid-40s. I gave up my career to raise my kids. My body has changed A LOT in recent years as I hit the roller coaster of perimenopause. I am a perfectionist who battles anxiety, crippling self-doubt, and a fear of failure. I don't love (or even like) a lot of those truths about myself, but they're not going anywhere. Instead of hating my body or resenting my husband for having a career when I don't or boxing myself in and never taking a risk so I can avoid failure, I've decided to do none of those things. Instead, I'm committed to doing the following:

- Keep learning about myself and figuring out skills and strategies to cope with my mental health struggles. That means I'm probably a "therapy for life" kind of girl because there will always be work to do.

- Work to actively stay out of my own way. That means taking scary risks, putting myself out there, and falling down and getting back up even when it's really, really hard.
- Find something positive to say about myself, to myself, every day.
- Continue to get stronger (mentally and physically) and distance myself from the toxic message that I need to be smaller or that my self-worth is tied to a number on a scale or on the tag of clothes.
- Foster positive relationships that fill me up. Also, recognize and walk away from toxicity.
- Rest, practice self-care, exercise, eat healthy foods, drink water (maybe someday 100 oz!), eat cake, drink wine, and live a life of joy in *this* body.
- Keep writing, keep talking to other women and mothers, and be honest about this journey of motherhood that is equal parts beautiful and heartbreaking at times.

And along the way, I'm going to figure it out. Whatever I'm going to be, whatever I'm going to do, when they've grown up and flown off to their own nests, it will become clear as I'm doing all of the things listed above.

I'm not going to compromise my own well-being by being a martyr.

I'm not going to try to be something I'm not (like the cool girl who looks effortlessly perfect on TV at a Packers game).

Whatever next-phase Karen is—stay at home in sweats Karen or go to work in Ann Taylor clothes Karen—she's still me. She's still awkward. She still talks too much. She still might choke on a sip of water and make a scene.

But most of all, the one thing I'll still be (even after they're gone) is Mom. And when one of them calls from college or from their first apartment to ask for advice on what to wear for a job interview or how to deal with a broken window or to tell me about a date they just had (and that this one might be the one!), I'll always answer. Even if my husband and I are on a 14-mile hike with our old-ass hips and knees.

Turtles apparently live forever, though, so my daughter better be taking those suckers with her when she goes.

---

## Notes on Chapter 30

*Whatever you end up doing when they grow up, don't ever compromise who you are.*
Learn about yourself, work on yourself, better what you can change and accept what you can't. Don't give up the things you love like '90s hip-hop or donuts on Sunday mornings, but remain open to trying new things too. Friend wants to take you to a metal concert? Why not? The waiter suggests the house special—a new food you've never tried? Check it out. You don't have to love it, but maybe you will.

And as for this next stage of your life, remember this. You've done a damn good job all these years as Mom. There's nothing you can't do.

# Epilogue

Well, that's it for now. I mean, I'm a wordy person and I probably have more to say (I never run out of things to say) but I'll wrap here. Hopefully, some of this helped if you're also lonely, or angry, or nervous about what comes next, or stressed about what to wear to a cocktail party in the winter when your inner body temp is locked in at 103 degrees.

If you take anything away from this book, please let it be this: Be kinder to yourself.

Give yourself grace and care and permission to rest.

Learn to accept that you're getting older and try to find appreciation for the body you're walking around in.

Gratitude is more powerful than most of us realize, so use it. Practice it.

When you're feeling frustrated that you went up a jeans size and super fit mom at school pickup doesn't ever seem to go up a jeans size, remember that she's dealing with shit too—I promise. Some of us just hide it better.

And don't hold back as you approach this next bend on the road of life. What do you want? You, who tucked all your hopes and dreams away in the back of the storage cabinet for all these years. What did eight-year-old you dream of being? Did she ever get there? Can she maybe get there now?

Don't let Guilt win.

Don't let the diet and anti-aging beauty industry win.

Live your life unapologetically. Laugh loudly, wear what you want to wear, invest in organic sheepskin oil neck masks or don't, but don't let anyone tell you you're less than if you have wrinkles or fat on your stomach or skin blotches or cellulite on your thighs.

We are so much more than our ages, our weight, or our clothing size—don't forget that.

If you're halfway there like I am, looking out at the view from atop the mountain, water your grass, soak in the view, and enjoy the descent. I plan on stopping along the way to travel the world with my husband and kids, have lots of girls' nights with wine and cheese dip, and pop into a coffee shop now and then to keep writing all of this down.

Maybe the next book will be *Good-Bye Periods! Grandma's in Menopause!* Stay tuned.

# Acknowledgments

This book was equal parts cathartic and heart wrenching to write, but I'm tremendously grateful for the opportunity. And I wouldn't have been able to do it without the help of so many influential and supportive people.

Thank you to Amy Fandrei, Sophie Thompson, and the rest of the team at Wiley. As a newbie, you were endlessly patient and instrumental in showing me the ropes of the book-writing process. Thank you for taking a chance on this book, taking a chance on me, and helping this vision come to life.

Thank you to the team at Smith Publicity for all your hard work in spreading the word about this book. (And for making me learn how to brag about myself that was tough, but a good experience and lesson for me.)

Thank you to Anabel Weeks for the professional hair and makeup photo shoot for my author bio and for making me feel like a glamorous movie star for a day. I don't know if I'll ever wear fake eyelashes again, but it was fun to try!

I'd like to send out a special thank you to Whitney Fleming for all of your support, guidance, and connections you've offered me—as both a fellow writer and as a friend. When I think about women who reach down to help other women who are coming up the ladder next, I think of you.

I also want to thank all of the writers and editors who have worked alongside me over the years. The online writing community is a strange world where you end up making best friends for life that you might never meet in person. But I appreciate all of you dearly, and each one of you has held a special place in my writing journey. There are too many names to list, but you know who you are.

The stories in this book are my own, but they are not without influence from other women and mothers in my life. I owe a debt of gratitude to my sister and my girlfriends for all your stories and unwavering support as I have navigated this writer-mom life. Thank you for showing up unexpectedly at my speaking events, sending me supportive texts and memes of encouragement, and even lending me your cabin for a weekend so I could escape to a quiet place to write. But mostly, thank you for saying things like "*You should write a book!*" and for defining true friendship in my life.

Thank you to my mom and dad for all the paper and pencils you endlessly handed me as kid so I could feed this dream. And to my husband and three children for giving me the space, time, and opportunity to put all of these words on paper. For believing in me. For letting me write about our little life. For bragging about me when I have struggled to brag about myself. And when people ask about me, thank you all for saying things like "My daughter?" or "My wife?" or "My mom?" and then "Oh, she's a writer." That validation means more than you know. I am where I am, doing what I love, because I have all of you in my corner.

To my partner for life, thank you for this beautiful journey and these amazing kids. What a story we've built. I love you all more than you know, even though you leave your stinky socks all over the house. I can't wait to see what adventures are coming next.

# About the Author

**Karen Johnson**, aka **The 21st Century SAHM**, is a former high school English teacher, turned stay-at-home-mom of three, turned writer, who lives in Wisconsin. Throughout her decades-long career in the online and in-print writing world, Karen has covered every parenting topic under the sun, from being an allergy mom to raising a strong-willed child to navigating the tumultuous ride of parenting teens. She has stood by her belief from the very beginning that we need humor to survive this crazy life of parenthood, and that we are all better mothers if we support one another.

Karen has essays featured in *Lose the Cape: Never Will I Ever (and then I had kids!)*, *The Unofficial Guide to Surviving Life with Boys: Hilarious and Heartwarming Stories About Raising Boys from the Boymom Squad*, and she is the author of *I Brushed My Hair Today: A Mom Journal for Mostly Together Moms*.

Karen's writing also has been featured on a long list of parenting websites including Scary Mommy, Parenting Teens and Tweens, Her View from Home, KC Parent Magazine, Today Parents, and Motherly, among others.

# About the Author

Karen graduated from College of the Holy Cross with a BA in English and Secondary Education. While a student at Holy Cross, Karen studied abroad for her entire junior year at the University of York in York, England. She later went on to earn an MA in Secondary Education from the University of Omaha.

Karen and her husband have hopped from state to state throughout their adult life, which means she taught high school English in Massachusetts, Nebraska, and Wisconsin before jumping into the SAHM life for eight years in Kansas and eventually moving back to Wisconsin. She's most grateful for this last move as living in a place with endless lakes, mild summers, and small bugs is her favorite.

When not sitting at her computer, Karen enjoys working out, walking her dog, and listening to podcasts about history, politics, or anything else that activates her brain cells. She's also an avid reader and loves to travel with her family. Because she has three busy kids (none of whom have their license yet) her other home is her beloved minivan that smells like hockey equipment and teenage angst.

You can find more information about Karen Johnson on her website the21stcenturysahm.com and find her on all social media as The 21st Century SAHM.